Ka Māno Wai

Ka Māno Wai

THE SOURCE OF LIFE

Noreen K. Mokuau,
S. Kukunaokalā Yoshimoto,
and Kathryn L. Braun

Photographs by
Shuzo Uemoto

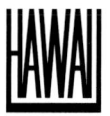

UNIVERSITY OF HAWAI'I PRESS
HONOLULU

Printed in China

First printing, 2023

Library of Congress Cataloging-in-Publication Data

Names: Mokuau, Noreen K., author. | Yoshimoto, S. Kukunaokalā, author. |
 Braun, Kathryn L., author. | Uemoto, Shuzo, photographer.
Title: Ka māno wai : the source of life / Noreen K. Mokuau, S.
 Kukunaokalā Yoshimoto and Kathryn L. Braun ; photographs by Shuzo
 Uemoto.
Other titles: Source of life
Description: Honolulu : University of Hawai'i Press, [2023] | Includes
 bibliographical references and index.
Identifiers: LCCN 2022047657 (print) | LCCN 2022047658 (ebook) | ISBN
 9780824894337 (Trade Paperback : acid-free paper) | ISBN 9780824893644
 (Hardback : acid-free paper) | ISBN 9780824894405 (pdf) | ISBN
 9780824894412 (epub) | ISBN 9780824894429 (Kindle Edition)
Subjects: LCSH: Elders (Indigenous leaders) —Hawaii. |
 Hawaiians—Intellectual life—Biography. | Culturally relevant
 pedagogy—Hawaii. | Hawaii—Biography.
Classification: LCC GR110.H38 M65 2023 (print) | LCC GR110.H38 (ebook) |
 DDC 398.209969—dc23/eng/20221227
LC record available at https://lccn.loc.gov/2022047657
LC ebook record available at https://lccn.loc.gov/2022047658.

Cover art: A stream in Waipao, He'eia, O'ahu. Photo by Shuzo Uemoto.

Designed by Mardee Melton

CONTENTS

PREFACE

Ua hoʻomaka mākou. We began. Our undertaking of *Ka Māno Wai: The Source of Life* started with a shared belief that Native Hawaiian ancestral practices can inform and advance health and social justice in Hawaiʻi. Our belief was underscored with an urgent and resolute commitment to preserve these practices by gathering moʻolelo (stories) of esteemed kumu loea (expert teachers) who are knowledge keepers of cultural ways. The kumu loea featured in this book are renowned cultural authorities in their specialty areas and are also our mentors, colleagues, friends, and family. Their specialty areas have origins in history, are deeply rooted in cultural worldviews and values, and are gently nuanced to reflect value for past, present, and future generations. The specialty areas are diverse, but all are anchored in the relational aspect of Hawaiian cosmography in which people, environment, and spirituality are intricately linked.

As Indigenous researchers and social scientists, our approach to gathering the moʻolelo of kumu loea placed the Native Hawaiian standpoint at the center. This approach prioritizes relational epistemology, which espouses that everything is related, interactive, and reciprocal. This approach also accords respect to cultural knowledge and recognizes story as a preferred method for gathering information. From 2018 to 2020, we individually met and talked story with thirteen kumu loea about their lives and cultural ʻike (knowledge) of ancestral practices. We utilized a short, open-ended, semistructured interview guide but allowed the kumu loea to direct the interview and to tell their stories as they unfolded for them. Their individual styles of sharing added to the richness of the information we received.

In their stories, kumu loea shared how family and their own kumu (teachers) guided their paths. They also identified historical and cultural resources from which they learned about cultural and practice traditions. We researched these resources and added this information to the chapters to complement the moʻolelo. For example, many kumu loea referred to ʻōlelo noʻeau (proverbs and poetical sayings). These proverbs were tools used in everyday life to transfer lessons from teacher to student and from kupuna (elder) to keiki (child). They provide insight into the thinking and worldview of Kānaka Maoli (Native Hawaiians), and are shared within moʻolelo to illustrate key points.

Initially, we met at least twice with each kumu loea, including a session with the photographer. As their stories were being written for chapters, kumu loea were engaged as reviewers who made corrections, offered suggestions, and gave us approval to move forward. We note the inclusion of Dr. Kekuni Blaisdell as a kumu loea (deceased 2016). He was a foremost authority on health among Native Hawaiians and is a beloved mentor. Written similarly to the other chapters, we have included a reprinted article on Dr. Blaisdell by three of his haumāna (students).

In keeping with an appreciation of the relational aspect of Native Hawaiian culture, we include photography of kumu loea in places that are uniquely meaningful to them. Most of the images are of kumu loea in the natural environment, but some kumu loea chose to be photographed in or outside their own homes or places of employment. The significance of place for most kumu loea is personal and distinctive, reflecting identity and a sense of belonging. Images are an artful medium that explicitly captures the visual context and implicitly captures the emotional connection of person and place. Natural environments that serve as the background for kumu loea include the Pacific Ocean, Nuʻuanu Park, Makiki Valley, Kaʻala Farm, Hāwea Heiau, Papahana Kuaola, and Ka Papa Loʻi O Kānewai.

We began with a belief in and a commitment to preserve ancestral practices that may advance health and social justice for Native Hawaiians and others. We used pule (prayer) liberally throughout our process to ensure that we were proceeding in a pono (correct, good, upright, in perfect order) manner and authentically reflecting the moʻolelo of kumu loea. Throughout the process, we deepened our appreciation for the role of these and all kumu loea in preserving, practicing, and transmitting Hawaiian knowledge. As we evolved in our understanding of Hawaiian culture, past and present, we gained new insights that will continue to inform our teaching, research, and service within the university system. We hope you will be inspired, as we were, by the stories of the kumu loea and will join us in continuing to search for cultural answers for health and social justice. E hoʻomau ana kākou. Let us persevere.

HOʻOMOE WAI KĀHI KE KĀOʻO.

Let all travel together like water flowing in one direction.

(PUKUI 1983, 118)

ACKNOWLEDGMENTS

Me ka mahalo palena ʻole (with gratitude beyond measure) we acknowledge the kumu loea (expert teachers) who have graciously shared ʻike kūhohonu (deep knowledge) on Kānaka (Native Hawaiians) cultural practices with us. Their stories are anchored in history, enriched with familial and personal experiences, and shape a future in which cultural practices can contribute to health and social justice. As knowledge keepers of Hawaiian culture, kumu loea are master practitioners and esteemed teachers who invest in improving health and justice for all people through their practice and teaching.

Me ka mahalo piha (with whole-hearted thankfulness) we acknowledge support from the Barbara Cox Anthony Endowment (BCA) in the Thompson School of Social Work & Public Health (TSSWPH). In line with the BCA mission to improve the lives of older adults in Hawaiʻi, this book highlights the wisdom of older adults regarding ancestral cultural practices that may benefit the diverse populations in our island homeland. We are also thankful to those who have supported our work with the numerous activities required in developing this book. We have benefited from the artistic talent of photographer Mr. Shuzo Uemoto, who captured the aloha and dignity of kumu loea with his beautiful pictures. We acknowledge the kākoʻo (support) of two graduate assistants. Mr. Tyran Terada, a doctoral candidate in social work, performed time-consuming activities such as interview transcription and glossary development. Ms. Keilyn Kawakami, a master's student in public health, provided invaluable kōkua (help) with glossary development, chapter and reference formatting, and overall technical support. We appreciate Ms. Theresa Kreif, assistant to the dean, and Mr. Keith Fujikawa, the administrative officer of TSSWPH, who facilitated our work with public relations and fiscal matters. We also want to thank Kamehameha Publishing for granting permission to reprint an article on Dr. Kekuni Blaisdell from *Hūlili: Multidisciplinary Research on Hawaiian Well-Being* and acknowledge the other authors of that article, Drs. Kamanaʻopono Crabbe and Kealoha Fox. The Hawaiʻi Pacific Foundation provides support to Native Hawaiian communities, and we recognize them for their generous support to the TSSWPH for educational curriculum that aligns with the themes of this book.

Me ka mahalo nui (with much thankfulness) we recognize the consistent guidance and support from the University of Hawaiʻi Press. Mahalo nui to Mr. Joel Cosseboom, former interim director and publisher, for his early conversations of encouragement and inspiration, to Ms. Emma Ching and Ms. Giannà Marsella for steady and invaluable asistance on editing and publishing, and to the entire UHP team for their meticulous care in helping us to complete our project.

Me ke aloha (with aloha) we recognize our families, who have stood with us throughout this journey. In particular, we wish to express our deep appreciation to kūpuna who have been our lifelong inspiration and guides, Norman and Angeline Mokuau, Sadie Carol Kealohilani Ayat, and Ruth Lenzner Braun. Also, we recognize our partners Frank Carlos Jr., Shy Kauanoe Helm, and Chris Conybeare for their abundance of care in keeping us grounded and helping us to soar at the same time. We acknowledge the incredible gifts that kumu loea have bestowed upon us with their precious time and stories, and we recognize our kuleana (responsibility, privilege) to transmit these stories in a manner that reflects the foundation of culture. Aloha aku, aloha mai. Aloha given, aloha received.

Noreen, Kukunaokalā, and Kathryn

CHAPTER 1

Hoʻomaka

In Native Hawaiian cosmography, the continuum of past, present, and future is fundamental to the identity of Kānaka (Native Hawaiians). One perspective in understanding Kānaka identity is through nā piko ʻekolu (three body points).

* The piko poʻo (head) is the connection to the past with the spiritual realm, including one's ʻaumākua (ancestors, family gods).
* The piko waena (umbilicus) is the connection to the present with parents and family.
* The piko maʻi (genitalia) is the connection to the infinite future through descendants. (Pukui, Haertig, and Lee 1972, 182–183)

Not only do the connections of the past, present, and future sustain Kānaka identity, they also perpetuate the ʻike (knowledge) of Native Hawaiian culture on health and social justice.

An ʻōlelo noʻeau (Hawaiian proverb and poetical saying) that captures the importance of our ancestors and ancestral past is:

I ULU NO KA LĀLĀ I KE KUMU.

The branches grow because of the trunk.

(Pukui 1983, 137)

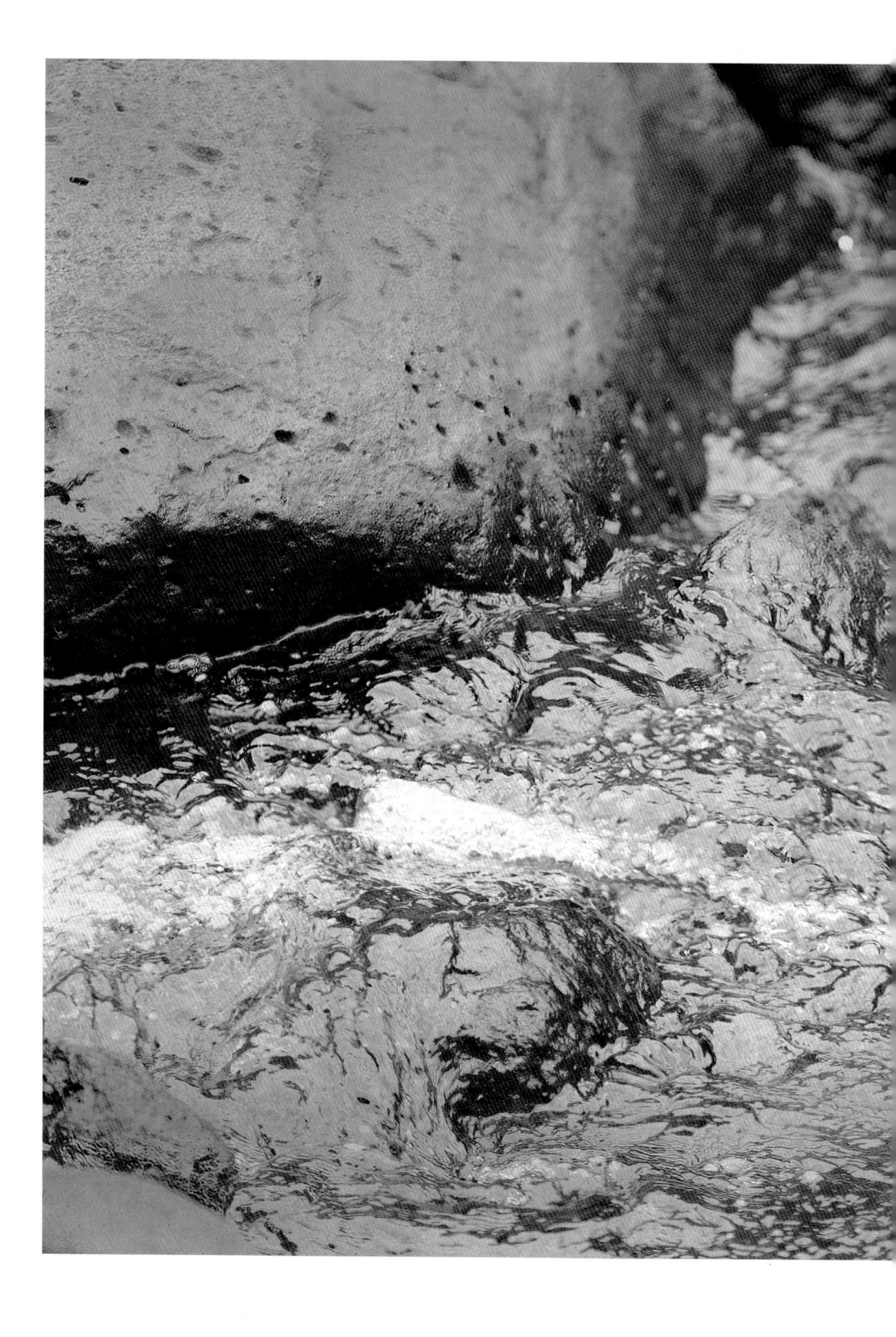

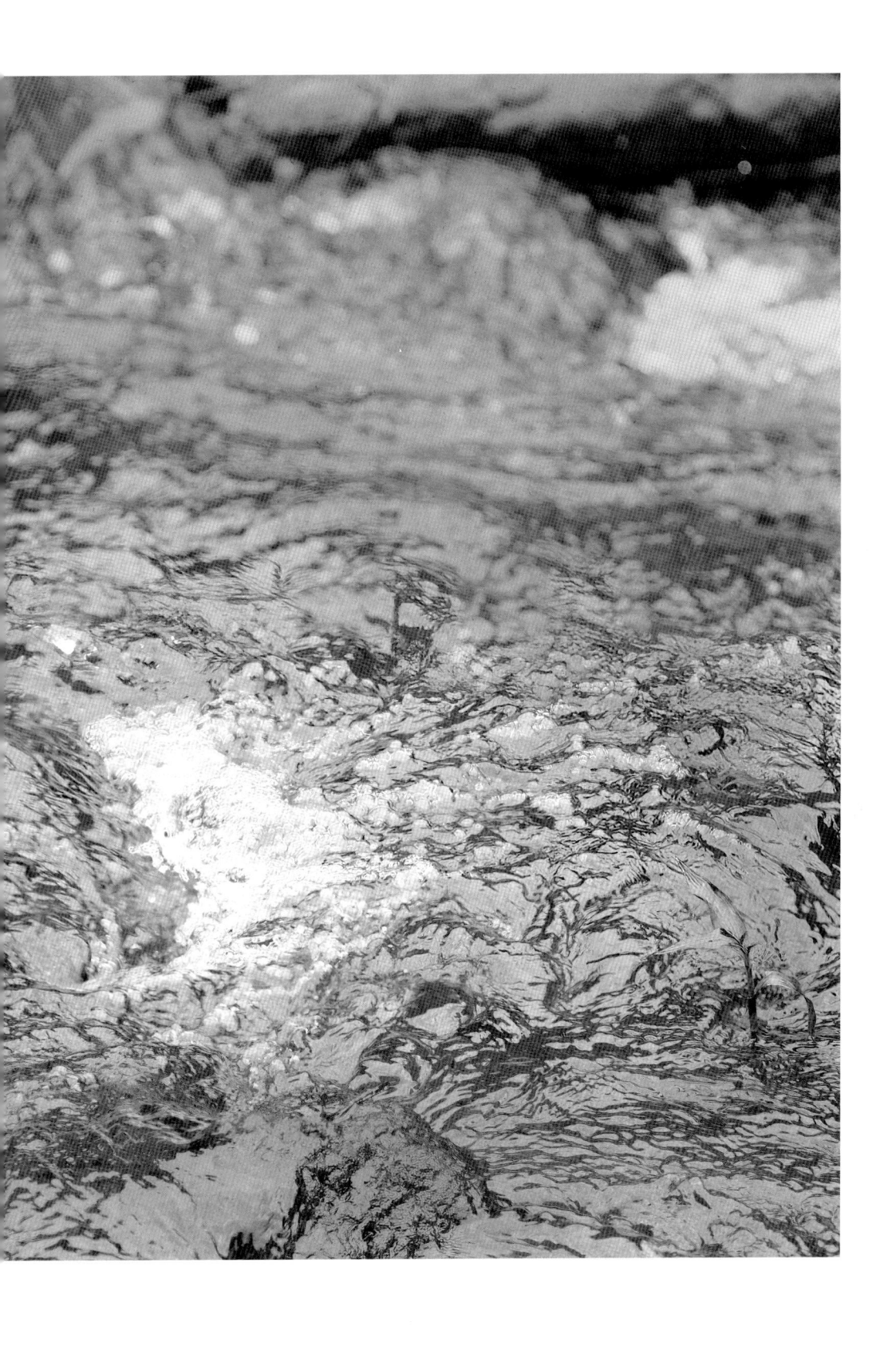

Ancestral Past

Historical accounts indicate that ancestral genealogies were rooted in spiritual worldviews that intricately linked the natural environment and people and ultimately shaped societal structure. Hawaiian societal structure had a defined government, divisions of people with specific roles, and sanctions and rituals around which life was organized (Ii 1983; Kamakau 1991; Malo 1951). Malo (1951) states that the government was supposed to have one body with the king as the head, the chiefs as the shoulders and chest, the kahuna o na kiʻi (high priest) as the right hand, the kanaka kālaimoku (chief counselor) as the left hand, the soldiery as the right foot, and the fishermen and farmers as the left foot (187). The makaʻāinana (commoners, populace) comprised the most numerous group of people. They were fixed residents of the land and contributed significantly to society as farmers, fishermen, house builders, and canoe makers. As the root word "ʻāina" denotes both "land" and "to eat," the phrase "makaʻāinana" describes the people who stewarded and lived on the land.

Life was organized around sanctions and rituals in order to establish the best relations with the gods (Malo 1951). There were cultural protocols with pule (prayer, prayers) and ceremonies for all aspects of living, including eating, fishing, farming, building shelters and canoes, and warfare. For example, ʻai kapu (system specifically regulating food and eating practices) denoted strong sanctions around eating. This included the separation of men and women in eating, and the restrictions that only men could cook food, and that women could not eat certain foods such as bananas. Religious tenets guided these sanctions, and deviation could result in death.

It is within this context of Hawaiian life that Westerners made contact in 1778. While there are various estimates of the Native Hawaiian census upon first contact with the West, conservative thinking of scholars suggests that the population was 250,000 to 300,000 people (Nordyke 1989). In historical records, Native Hawaiians were viewed as a thriving and robust people, with "extraordinary muscular development, in women as well as men" that reflected their "vigorous and strenuous outdoor existence" (Snow 1974, 11).

Yet by 1850, the Native Hawaiian population had decreased to approximately 84,000 people, a dramatic decline of more than 70 percent (Nordyke 1989). The most significant cause of depopulation was the introduction of infectious diseases by foreigners, including measles, tuberculosis, smallpox, and syphilis.

With depopulation came the dismantling of Hawaiian culture, as Western contact increased, with missionaries and others settling in Hawaiʻi. The dismantling can be observed in three historic "events" with tumultuous consequences: (a) the introduction of Christianity; (b) the alteration of the land system through the mahele (division); and (c) the overthrow of the Hawaiian monarchy (Mokuau and Matsuoka 1995). The Hawaiian worldview, in which spirituality permeated all aspects of life, was replaced by a fundamentally different Christian perspective in 1820. The Christian perspective altered the Kānaka life, as the multitude of Hawaiian gods were replaced by one god, the use of the Hawaiian language was supplanted with English, and customary traditions, such as the hula (dance), were discouraged. Along with these cosmographic and structural changes, the system of land control and ownership was altered. Under the mahele in 1848, there was a significant loss of lands, and the majority of Hawaiians became disposed of land and resources, while foreign landownership quickly escalated (Kameʻeleihiwa 1992; Van Dyke 2008). By the end of the nineteenth century, White men owned four acres of land for every one owned by a Native (Daws 1974). The culmination of foreign influence resulted in the orchestrated overthrow of the Hawaiian monarchy by the United States in 1893, with Hawaiʻi being annexed in 1898 and then becoming a territory.

The historical impact of cultural losses on Native Hawaiians is evident today, as there is an excess burden of health and social disparities. "Historical trauma" has been defined as the cumulative emotional and psychological wounding over the life span and across generations, emanating from massive group trauma (Brave Heart 2000). Analysis of trauma includes an examination of physical, economic, cultural, social, and psychological impacts (Wesley-Esquimaux and Smolewski 2004) and has relevance for indigenous peoples such as Native Hawaiians (Braun et al. 2014; Goebert et al. 2018; Mokuau and Mataira 2013). In Hawaiʻi, Native Hawaiians have the shortest life expectancy and exhibit higher mortality rates than the total population due to heart disease, cancer, stroke, and diabetes (Mokuau et al. 2016; Wu et al. 2017). Poor health is inextricably linked to socioeconomic factors, and Native Hawaiians are more likely to live below the poverty level and have higher rates of unemployment and imprisonment (Office of Hawaiian Affairs 2010). Noteworthy and disturbing is the high percentage of Native Hawaiians who are without homes in their own island homeland (Yamane, Oeser, and Omori 2010).

Despite a historic downward trajectory in the quality of health and social conditions for Native Hawaiians, there is also evidence of resiliency (Antonio et al. 2020; Browne, Mokuau, and Braun 2009; Carlton et al. 2006). Resilience focuses on protective and recovery factors and draws from the strengths perspective that recognizes the inherent power of individuals and communities (Saleebey 1997). For many Native Hawaiians, resiliency is anchored in the ways of the ancestral past. There is a growing body of information that promotes the use of culturally anchored solutions, along with non-Native best-practice interventions, to restore health and improve social justice (Braun et al. 2021; Kaholokula, Nacapoy, and Dang 2009; Mokuau, Braun, and Daniggelis 2012; Tsark, Blaisdell, and Aluli 1998). Drawing upon the powerful values and practices of old Hawaiʻi may contribute to the resolution of health and social disparities for present and future generations.

Kumu Loea as Sources of Knowledge

One way to learn about ancestral solutions for health and social justice is through the moʻolelo (stories) of kumu loea (expert teachers). The kumu who shared their stories in this book are knowledge keepers of Hawaiian culture. They contribute to the preservation and perpetuation of Hawaiian culture through their practice and teaching of specialty areas that are grounded in ancestral ways. As sources of wisdom of cultural knowledge and skills, they hold the answers to the connections of the past, present, and future. An ʻōlelo noʻeau that captures this sentiment is:

KA POUHANA.

The main post.

(PUKUI 1983, 167)

Kumu loea are knowledgeable in diverse specialty areas that have relevance for health and social justice. All of these areas embrace the relational aspects of people, the environment, and the spiritual realm. Highlights of their stories are provided below.

* Mana (spiritual, supernatural, or divine power) is fundamental to Kānaka culture. Hawaiian edict suggests mana can be viewed as both hereditary and

acquired and can be enhanced or diminished. Dr. Kamanaʻopono Crabbe discusses mana as being central to the Hawaiian worldview and draws implications for contemporary society.

* Mālama kūpuna (care for elders and ancestors) and mālama ʻāina (care for the land) are areas of great significance for Kānaka. In acknowledging the clear connections of people and land, Ms. Linda Paik addresses the repatriation and the respectful reburial of Native Hawaiian ancestors and caring for sacred lands as ways to perpetuate culture.

* ʻĀina momona (fertile, fruitful land, and ocean) refers to the abundance of the land and ocean nourishing people through careful stewardship. Mr. Eric Enos describes the urgency of caring for the land as a source of cultural identity, cultural safety, and rich food sources.

* ʻAi (to eat, food) sustains health and contributes to a thriving population. In an island ecosystem such as Hawaiʻi, people in traditional times were reliant on the land and ocean to support the practice of ʻaiola (to eat nutritious foods). Dr. Claire Hughes addresses traditional practices associated with food and discusses the advantages of the Hawaiian diet for people today.

* ʻŌlelo (language) uniquely identifies a group of people. The importance of the Kānaka language is amplified in context of its genesis in an oral-auditory tradition. Ms. Sarah Keahi speaks about the cherished value of the Hawaiian language and the need to perpetuate its use as a vehicle to promote Hawaiian culture.

* Mele (song, songs) of contemporary times are the poetic expression of ideas through words and melody. While this is different from the vocal expressions of traditional Hawaiʻi, the meanings of mele have connections to culture. Dr. Jonathan Osorio describes the uses of mele and underscores the value of mele in advocacy and social justice.

* Hoʻoponopono (setting to right, the process of conflict resolution) is deeply anchored in Hawaiian culture as a means to resolve family conflict. Mrs. Lynette Paglinawan delineates the context and steps of hoʻoponopono and proclaims its usefulness in dealing with the complex array of issues confronting people and families in contemporary society.

* Lāʻau lapaʻau (Hawaiian medicinal plants) is the traditional practice of using plants, minerals, and prayer to restore health. Ms. Leinaʻala Bright describes how she incorporates lāʻau lapaʻau into her healing practice, and how she is working to integrate traditional Hawaiian healing practices into home settings and health clinics.

- Lomilomi (to rub, press, knead, massage) is a traditional healing practice that restores health through physical manipulation of the body using the hands, arms, knees, feet, and even sticks. Mr. Keola Chan explains the origins and techniques of lomilomi and espouses its potential for helping people deal with health problems.

- Kaula (cordage and rope) was an essential component in traditional Kānaka culture. It was used in daily activities such as the construction of houses, the building of canoes, the securing of food, and the making of weapons. ʻŌlohe lua (lua master) Sonny Kaulukukui expounds on the cultivation, preparation, and uses of kaula, and emphasizes its value for cultural identity and esteem today.

- Lua (Hawaiian art of fighting) is the fighting style of formidable expert warriors in traditional times. This form of fighting pre-existed King Kamehameha I by more than two centuries and was characterized by hand-to-hand combat. ʻŌlohe lua Jerry Walker discusses the history, practice, and significance of lua today.

- Nā mea kaua (Hawaiian weapons) are the armaments that supported the hand-to-hand fighting of Kānaka warriors. The weapons were made of natural products and intended to inflict harm when people were within striking distance. ʻŌlohe lua ʻUmi Kai reports on weaponry and its implications for the preservation of culture and identity.

- Native Hawaiian law is that distinctive area that acknowledges Native Hawaiians as Indigenous peoples with unique and distinct rights. Attorney Melody MacKenzie provides a definitive perspective on social justice and critical legal issues for Native Hawaiians, with attention to public land trust.

- An icon in Native Hawaiian health is physician Dr. Kekuni Blaisdell (deceased 2016), who taught generations of medical students and mentored numerous other advocates in health equity and social justice. In a reprinted article from Kamehameha Publishing, three of his haumāna (students)—Drs. Noreen Mokuau, Kamanaʻopono Crabbe, and Kealoha Fox—share personal stories of his vision and influence.

Knowledge Keepers

As knowledge keepers of Hawaiian culture, kumu loea are master practitioners and esteemed teachers. They exhibit a strong commitment to helping Hawaiians and all people through practice and teaching. They are clear that historical trauma contributed to disparities experienced by Native Hawaiians today and are ambitious in their desire to prevent further erosion of cultural identity and well-being.

As master practitioners, they are disciplined in specialty areas that have origins in Hawaiian culture. For example, some kumu loea focus on reclaiming health through eating nutritious foods from a traditional Hawaiian diet and caring for a bountiful land that will nourish and sustain people. Others engage in healing practices such as lomilomi, lā'au lapa'au, and ho'oponopono. Others advocate for social justice through mele and law. They are convinced that drawing on ancestral practices can lead to the building of cultural esteem, worth, and identity. These practices can help improve health and well-being and contribute to social justice for present and future generations.

The kumu loea are cultural leaders who are dedicated to the teaching of others. Their sources of knowledge are inherited and acquired and include ancestral and living teachers. They have all shared the genealogy of their practice, expressing deep appreciation for their own teachers. Further, they learn through observation, modeling, and practice in classrooms in the natural environment and in buildings. Their commitment to teaching others is balanced with their lifelong seeking of knowledge to ensure their own continual learning, and is reflected in this 'ōlelo no'eau:

E HANA MUA A PA'A KE KAHUA MAMUA O KE A'O ANA AKU IA HA'I.

Build yourself a firm foundation before teaching others.

(PUKUI 1983, 34)

Common Themes

The mo'olelo of kumu loea poignantly address the central premise of this book: that ancestral practices hold value for health and social justice for present and future generations. Kumu loea are unique and distinctive, and no two stories are exactly alike, yet common themes that build the premise of this book emerge across the chapters. As you read this book, we draw your attention to several themes that enrich individual chapters and have added value across chapters.

First, kumu loea discussed rich historical and cultural antecedents, highlighting the pilina (relationship) of spirituality, environment, and people, as they related to the origins and practice of their specialty areas. Strict spiritual customs involving prayers, invocations, rituals, and ceremonial preparations were associated with all specialty areas, and mana is inherent in all practices guided by spiritual standards. While kumu loea did not speak directly to "holding mana" themselves, they referred in their mo'olelo to the importance of spiritual power in both the practitioner and the practice. Mana has transformative value when infused and shared by kumu loea in practices that deal with health and social justice. For the practitioner, mana could be inherited through genealogy and connections, but it could also be acquired from teachers and experts who led in different domains of knowledge and through practice (Crabbe, Fox, and Coleman 2017). Readers can learn from the manner in which kumu loea express and share mana as a means to heal, restore resiliency, and resolve social injustices.

Second, kumu loea attributed importance to the sense of place. These places were most typically related to personal and family geography, such as ancestral homes or communities where one was raised. For example, simple statements such as "I am from Hilo" or "I come from Ho'olehua" yielded rich information on their family, lineage, and community. Kumu loea also spoke of wahi pana (legendary places) associated with significant legends, landmarks, and historical events. In acknowledging the importance of place, kumu loea shared stories that connected their activities and teachings to natural cultural settings such as the lo'i (irrigated taro terrace), the forest, and the ocean: "In the Hawaiian mind, a sense of place was inseparably linked with self-identity and self-esteem" and emphasized the land, ocean, and sky as living entities (Kanahele 1986, 188). Readers will be able to understand how kumu loea signify the importance of place in their development as practitioners and in their practice.

Third, kumu loea collectively viewed genealogy and family as central to their identity and growth. Kumu loea have roots in their families, and their families have roots in ancestral and family places. Many kumu loea were able to trace paternal and maternal 'ohana (family) across several generations, recounting the places they lived and the work they did. Several kumu loea had a parent who experienced being hānai (fostered, adopted), and spoke easily about the open, informal kinship system in Hawaiian families. In these situations, the hānai child was ho'okama (loved and treated as one's own) (Handy and Pukui 1972). It was not unusual for the child and

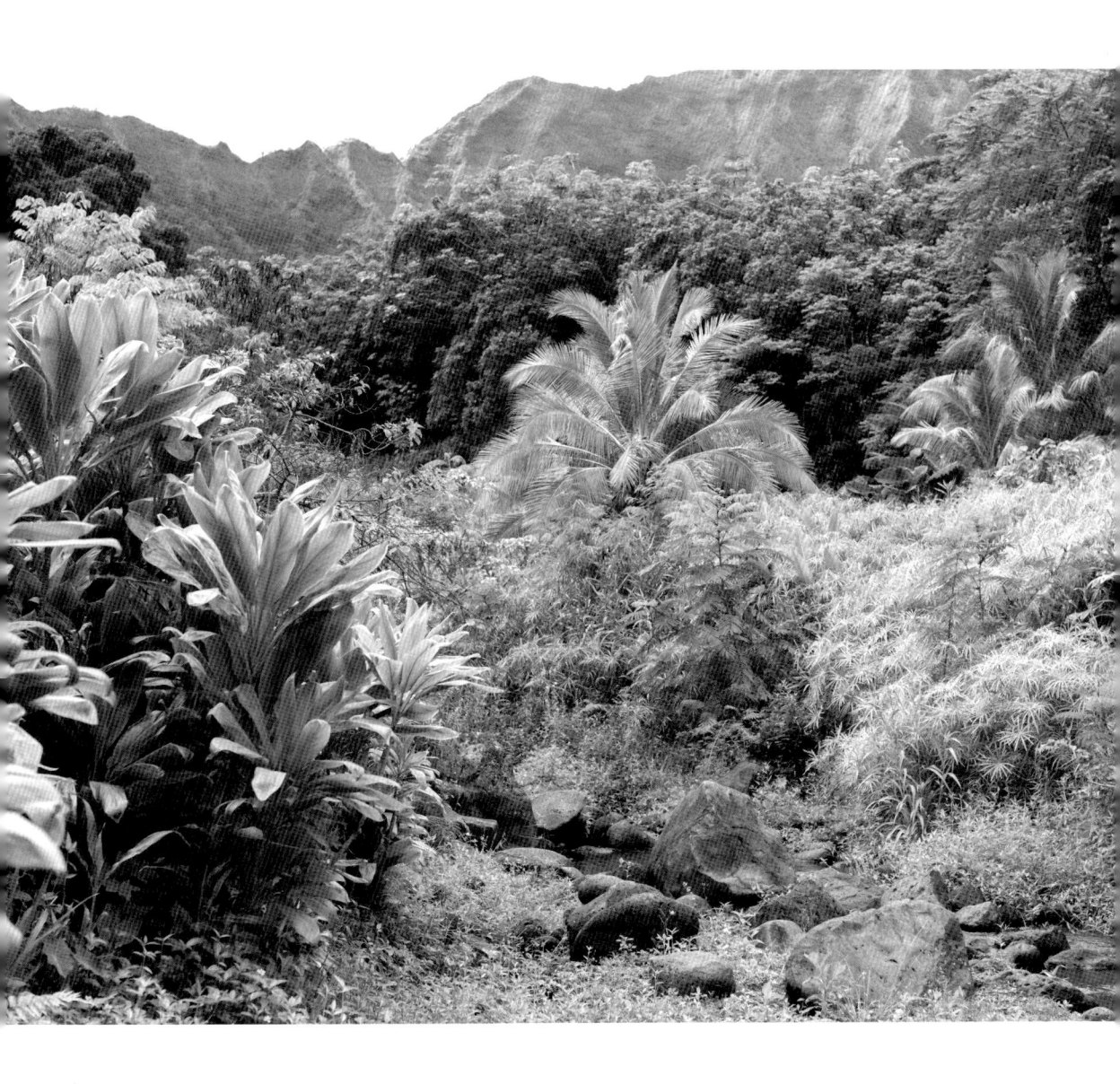

hānai family to maintain contact with the child's biological family. A few kumu loea were given special inoa (names) that held mana and conveyed particular meanings. A Hawaiian name might tell of the place or condition of birth, reveal lineage, identify the ancestor's occupation, define social distinction, or allude to personal or family qualities (Pukui et al. 1979). Those kumu loea with special inoa admitted to a kuleana (responsibility, privilege) in holding values and behaviors that would accord respect to their names.

Readers will begin to appreciate the varying degrees of familial influence on the development and positions of kumu loea.

Fourth, readers will note the use of 'ōlelo Hawai'i (Hawaiian language) and 'ōlelo no'eau in all chapters. The interweaving of the Hawaiian language provides the reader with a foundational understanding of Hawaiian ways of knowing, thinking, and being. The 'ōlelo no'eau were shared to enhance knowledge of the language as seen through the lens of ancestral practices and relevant to health and social justice. While the proficiency and usage comfortability levels differed for each kumu loea, all incorporated the Hawaiian language into their story.

Fifth, all kumu loea demonstrated a humility about their expertise, attributing their skills to akua (gods), their family, their kumu, their colleagues, and their haumāna. They spoke with humility and generosity, even as they showed themselves to be authoritative experts in their respective areas. In Hawaiian society, qualities of leadership such as lokomaika'i (generosity) and aloha (love, affection, compassion) were well recognized (Kanahele 1986). Kumu loea demonstrated these qualities. Readers are reminded that with colonization, efforts were made to erase and minimize many of these cultural practices. In this context, the kumu loea in this book, their teachers, and their teachers' teachers are courageous leaders who demonstrate a fierceness in perpetuating cultural practices.

Lastly, all kumu describe how they learned and perpetuated their practices, and readers will discern the multiple and complex forms of knowledge in Hawaiian culture. Kumu loea recognized value in many non-Native approaches to health and social justice, and several appreciated efforts to integrate Native and non-Native approaches depending on the individual, family, and community context. Kumu loea demonstrated an ardent commitment to their specialty areas, but they emphasized that there were many Native Hawaiians who held cultural 'ike and acknowledged different approaches and styles of practice. They would say "Others may do it differently but this is the way I learned" or "This is the way I was taught." In saying this, they reminded us to be open and appreciative of the diverse ways of knowing.

'A'OHE PAU KA 'IKE I KA HĀLAU HO'OKĀHI.

All knowledge is not taught in the same school.

(PUKUI 1983, 24)

They also recognized that, over time, historical practices appropriate for past generations may not be fully useful today. The relevance of ancestral practices occurs through thoughtful adaptation that responds to present-day health and social justice realities. For example, some kumu loea specifically indicated that students did not have to subscribe to the spiritual tenets of the specialty area but must be respectful of the spiritual foundation. Readers will note the ways that kumu loea maintained the authenticity of ancestral practices while still making modifications for the current context of Hawaiʻi and Hawaiians.

Panina (Closing)

The collective moʻolelo of these kumu loea promote the perpetuation of Kānaka ancestral practices. The title of this book, *Ka Māno Wai: The Source of Life,* has multilayered meanings. The literal definition, "source of water and of life; heart and circulatory system," acknowledges the vital importance of wai (fresh water) to sustaining life.

Before the arrival of Westerners in 1778, water was recognized as the source of all life in Hawaiʻi. Continuous mauka to makai (from the mountains to the oceans) stream flow was critical to providing fresh water for drinking, supporting traditional agriculture and aquaculture, recharging groundwater supplies, and supporting productive estuaries and fisheries by both bringing nutrients from the uplands to the sea and maintaining a travel corridor through which native stream animals could migrate between the streams and ocean to complete their life cycles (Sproat 2015, 526).

Figurative meanings encompass the nuances of cultural values and beliefs. Recognized as one of the most important elements on earth, water holds deep cultural and spiritual significance to Native Hawaiians. Water is viewed as a physical manifestation of Kāne (Hawaiian God), who is recognized as giving life to humankind and Earth (Kanahele 1986). As a natural resource, wai is central to Hawaiian cosmology, in which there is a spiritual foundation and an interconnectedness and interdependence of land, air, and water. One example of its significance can be seen when the word wai is repeated: "Waiwai is the Hawaiian word for wealth" (364). As a precious resource, we view water as symbolic of ancestral practices. In the same manner that water can sustain life, so can ancestral practices. Ancestral practices are anchored in Hawaiian cosmography and circulate as the foundation of culture. As such, these practices may bring promise to improved health and social justice for Native Hawaiians and for all who are inspired to follow these ways.

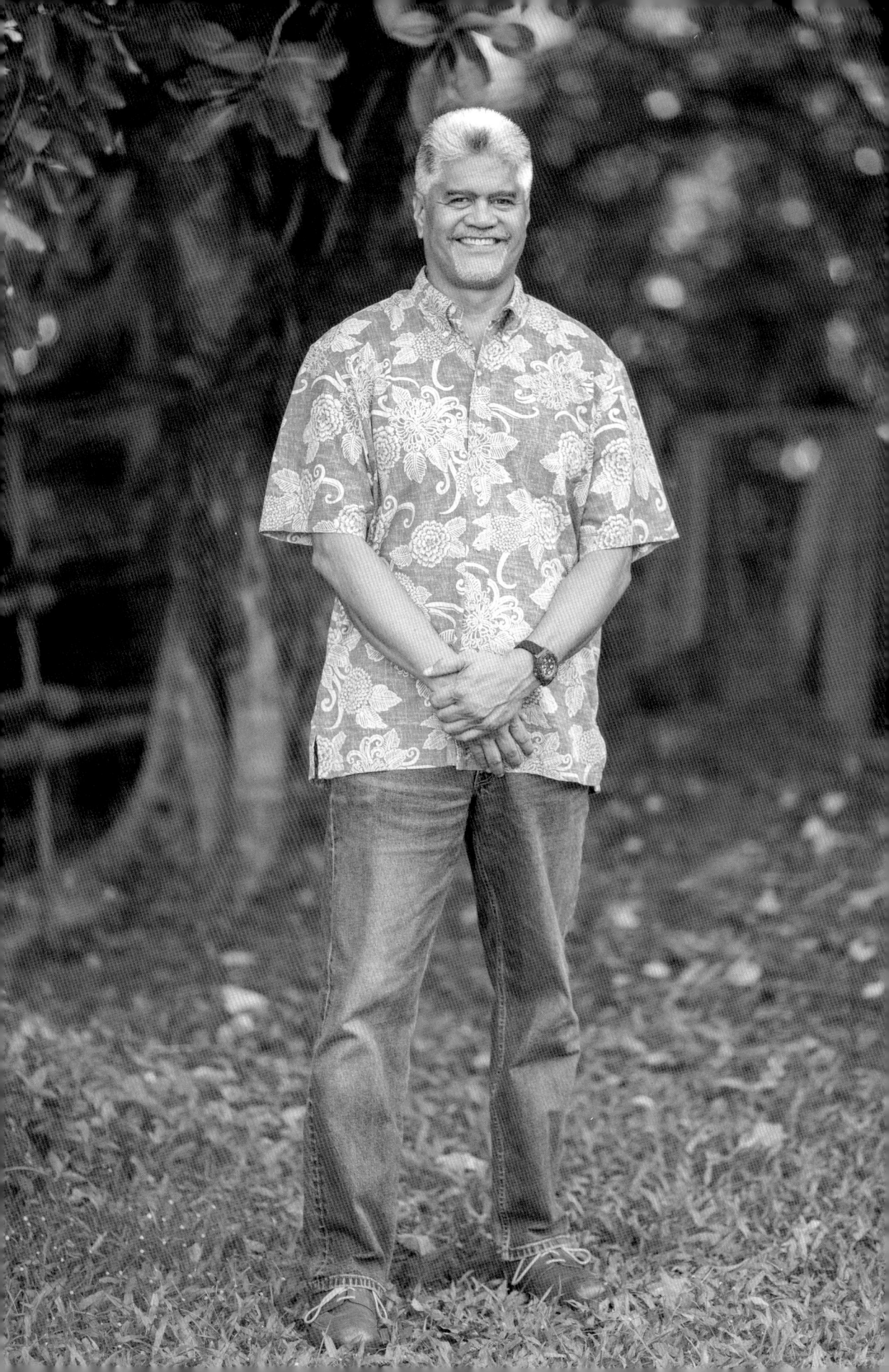

CHAPTER 2

Kamanaʻopono M. Crabbe

MANA

The Hawaiian dictionary defines "mana" as "spiritual, supernatural, or divine power," but as with many Hawaiian words, there is really no English translation that fully captures its meaning and significance for Native Hawaiians (Crabbe, Fox, and Coleman 2017). Scholars agree that you cannot understand the Polynesian worldview without an understanding of mana (Shore 1989). "Mana has been an elusive spiritual path I've been trying to understand throughout my lifetime," says Dr. Kamanaʻopono M. Crabbe. "It has been an important belief in my personal journey and professional career, and I believe mana is a central component of contemporary Native Hawaiian identity."

As the research director (2010–2012) and the Ka Pouhana–CEO (2012–2019) of the Office of Hawaiian Affairs (OHA), Kamanaʻopono, also known as Kamanaʻo, initiated a project to explore traditional and contemporary concepts of mana. Over several years, he and the OHA research staff consolidated information on mana from writings of Hawaiian scholars, ʻōlelo noʻeau, Hawaiian-language nūpepa (newspapers), and focus groups. The final product was a much-acclaimed book, *Mana Lāhui Kānaka,* which provides a discourse that more fully articulates the context and complexity of mana for Native Hawaiians (Crabbe, Fox, and Coleman 2017).

Kamanaʻo describes mana as a concept, a belief, and a philosophy that originates in the spiritual and cosmological realms and is reflected in the physical and the living realms. "For Native Hawaiians, our mana depends on balancing what we know is pono (correct, good, upright, in perfect order) with our kuleana as Kānaka ʻōiwi (Native peoples). Much of the foundation of ancient Hawaiian spirituality and morality consisted of the mediation, nego-tiation, and actualization of pono and kuleana in daily life, with respect to their effects on the mana of kānaka" (Crabbe, Fox, and Coleman 2017).

Mana Lāhui Kānaka provides evidence from historical records and scholars that Native Hawaiians believed in two sources of mana—mana that was inherited genealogically and mana that was acquired through belief or practice—although there was likely to be interplay between these sources (Pukui, Haertig, and Lee 1972). "We can start by saying mana is spiritual in the sense it is the lifestyle you live and the path you walk to be pono," says Kamana'o. "It can be inherited and acquired. But when I talk about mana with others, it is sometimes easiest to illustrate with examples from my life."

Mo'okū'auhau and Inherited Mana

Kamana'o's mother was Rose Na'auao "Maka" Pelayo, and her grandpar-ents were Solomon Kana'auao-Huewa'a and Julia Kawaikaunu of Kīpahulu, Kakalahale-Wailamoa, on Maui. The Kana'auao-Huewa'a clan included priests associated with voyaging, fishing, and canoeing, and the family line traces back to seafarers named after the star constellation Makali'i (the Ple-iades) that rises during Makahiki (a time of thanksgiving and ceremonial competition). The Kawaikaunu line included well-known lau hala (panda-nus leaf) weavers with their own special patterns. "At the last family reunion in July 2018," says Kamana'o, "we reviewed our mo'okū'auhau [genealogy], and we identified around 2,300 descendants from our great-grandparents."

His father, Mogul Kaleokalanakila (Lei of Victory) Crabbe, was the grandson of Horace Kalawai'a of Coconut Grove, Ko'olaupoko, O'ahu. When Kamana'o's great-grandfather, Horace, moved to Honolulu for school in the mid-1800s, he was hānai by two brothers with the surname Crabbe from Scotland who served the government of the Kingdom of Hawai'i. "My grandfather, father, and his 'ohana kept the name Crabbe to honor the men who cared for my great-grandfather. We acknowledged their roots, as well as our ancestral lineage as descendants of Kalawai'a."

Kamana'o grew up in two worlds. While there was a push by his grand-parents and parents to excel in the Western educational system, his grand-parents were native speakers of 'ōlelo Hawai'i, and the family lifestyle was very Hawaiian. The family would fish together and go crabbing, and pick 'opihi (limpet), wana (sea urchin), and limu kala (seaweed) from the oceans.

His family would spend time in the countryside. They would attend lūʻau (Hawaiian feasts) to celebrate a baby's first birthday or a wedding or to participate in a funeral. Kamanaʻo remembers, "I was on this path since I was young because my mom's family was of the generation that was transitioning from old to contemporary Hawaiʻi."

"My granduncle, Robert Kahoʻokele Naʻauao, in many ways exemplified mana, with his physical stature, strong principles and values, and cultural knowledge and behaviors. He was a big man, six foot, four inches, and he had a commanding presence," says Kamanaʻo. Uncle Bob came to Honolulu from Kīpahulu after his parents died. He arrived barefoot in Honolulu harbor with a bag of clothes and some food, and he spoke no English, only ʻōlelo Hawaiʻi. Honolulu was a new world to him, filled with haole (Caucasian) and Asian people. But he adjusted well. He became a star athlete in football and basketball at McKinley High School. Later, he was one of Hawaiʻi's first Aloha Week kings. He took up a career in corrections and went on to become the chief warden at Oʻahu Community Correctional Center. Adds Kamanaʻo, "He helped me a lot as I was growing up. I describe him as a bigger, brawnier version of Duke Kahanamoku."

Kamanaʻo remembers his childhood as a good one. "But in high school and in my early twenties, I was quite kolohe (wild, mischievous)." He moved to San Francisco after high school and served in the army reserves, training in South Carolina and Georgia. He remembers partying a lot. "But I realized at that time that wasn't where I needed to be. So I came back home, and my mom said, 'You're going to go to Uncle Bob.' So I kind of was hānai by him." It was with Uncle Bob that Kamanaʻo started his deep learning about his heritage. Kamanaʻo would go to his uncle's house to help clean the house or the yard. While he was there, Uncle Bob would share about the Kanaʻauao-Huewaʻa family genealogy and ancestors, about the traditional way of life he experienced growing up in Kīpahulu, and about life in general. Adds Kamanaʻo, "At the same time, I was taking Hawaiian language at Kapiʻolani Community College and I would practice by conversing with Uncle Bob in ʻōlelo Hawaiʻi."

Kamanaʻo learned about inherited mana by learning his own moʻokūʻauhau. He says,

> It took years to get to the point where I can recite my lineage back to a minimum of six generations and describe my kūpuna's ʻāina hānau [birthplace] in detail. For example, my great-grandparents come from

Kīpahulu, Maui. The wind there is Ka Makanikaʻilialoha, the peak is called Palikea . . . it's on the back of Haleakalā and shrouded in mist. The wailele [waterfall] in the back valley is named Waimoku, and it cascades down to the kahawai [river, freshwater ecosystems, and streams] of ʻOheo. The bay is called Kukui, and Puhilele is the peninsula where the blowhole spouts upward. Kanekauilanuimakehaikalani is the heiau [spiritual site], which was used for stargazing and aligning stars, which pairs up with my family's history of navigation, canoeing, [and] voyaging. I can talk about my family heritage now, but it took my granduncle to share this with me in a way that helped me get back on my own path.

Knowing one's moʻokūʻauhau allowed Hawaiians to trace the origins of their lineage and mana to the ancestral gods. Moʻokūʻauhau recorded the accumulation of mana over generations and were themselves considered sacred because of the mana they carried (Crabbe, Fox, and Coleman 2017). "We often think of this as mana akua, which translates as 'mana from the gods,'" says Kamanaʻo. Prior to contact with the West, the mōʻī (monarch) or aliʻi (chief, chiefs) would go into the ʻanuʻu tower (raised place) at the heiau during certain times of the year, for example, when the sun was directly overhead. "When the light from the sun goes into the tower, the mōʻī or aliʻi would receive mana akua," Kamanaʻo said.

The oli (chant) known as Mele a Pākui (chant of the ancient gods and lineages of early chiefs in Hawaiʻi) relays the story of Wākea (ancestor of the Hawaiian people) and Papa (ancestor of the Hawaiian people) and the formation of the Hawaiian Islands. But this oli also recounts the early progenitors of chiefly lines. For example, one of the paramount chiefly lines came from Laʻamaikahiki. He had three sons, triplets born on the same day from different mothers. One child grew up to be the chiefly line for Kauaʻi, another for Oʻahu, and the third for Maui. "So the chant records the mana akua to the mana aliʻi, but it's through genealogy," says Kamanaʻo. The mōʻī, but especially King Kalākaua and King Kauikeaouli (Kamehameha III), would consult the kahuna moʻokūʻauhau (expert in genealogy) regarding various mele koʻihonua (cosmogonic genealogical chants). The kings then could understand an individual's inherited mana and his or her standing, rank, authority, and genealogical links.

Acquired Mana

In addition to recognizing that mana was inherited by individuals through moʻokūʻauhau, Kānaka believed that mana could be "enhanced, acquired, amplified, diminished, or lost through a range of actions that were either aligned with or counter to socio-cultural and spiritual understanding of proper behaviors" (Crabbe, Fox, and Coleman 2017, 37). Says Kamanaʻo, "So another way to mana is through formal training. You acquire mana as you learn pule, you learn oli, you learn how to conduct ritual and ceremony. As you are doing this, mana is being created. When you go through formal Hawaiian knowledge acquisition, and when you learn to apply it, that's acquired mana."

Kamanaʻo undertook such training himself by studying ritual and ceremony from kumu (teacher) Hokulani Holt-Padilla. As part of this training, Kamanaʻo learned to chant the 127-line Mele Koʻihonua, a genealogical chant that describes various characteristics or traits of the people involved in a particular genealogy. "But in order to learn ritual and ceremony, you need to learn a whole body of knowledge, belief systems, protocols, and cultural references to help you develop a keen sense of good critical thinking, etiquette, and mannerisms. You've got to learn about your environment, the wind, the stars, the ocean currents," says Kamanaʻo. This is because certain places have mana and therefore can impart such mana, particularly places that are consecrated or kapu (taboo) for specific spiritual purposes (Crabbe, Fox, and Coleman 2017). As well as studying ritual and ceremony, Kamanaʻo studied lua, hoʻoponopono, and ʻawa ceremony (a ceremony in which a drink from the kava plant is prepared, passed, and sipped as a sign of commitment to things Hawaiian).

While Kamanaʻo was studying with kumu Holt-Padilla and other kumu, he also was pursuing his master's and doctoral degrees in psychology from the University of Hawaiʻi to learn Western concepts of behavior and research. He remembers:

> It was hard to do both, but I found that the chanting and the ceremony, going to Hana on Maui, wearing malo [the traditional Hawaiian loincloth], and chanting as the Hōkūleʻa [contemporary Hawaiian voyaging canoe] sailed into Hana Bay provided an essential balance. I needed that to help replenish my motivation to be in

school. I found my own way to balance both because I knew that my cultural training was a source of strength and a source of mana to help me accomplish what I needed to do at the university.

In Hawaiian society, experts in every field were respected and considered to have great mana. Some inherited this mana through their lineage. But they also needed to thoroughly acquire the knowledge and skills of their field and apply them to enhance and increase their mana. "Education and mentoring were not only important means of passing on traditional knowledge, but also were a highly spiritual process that allowed Kānaka to gradually acquire mana" (Crabbe, Fox, and Coleman 2017, 41). This gave Native Hawaiians access to mana and allowed Native Hawaiians to acquire mana regardless of their genealogical status. The following ʻōlelo noʻeau speaks to acquired mana:

MA KA HANA KA ʻIKE.

In working one learns.

(PUKUI 1983, 227)

The historical record also notes that "failing to act in pono ways or failing to fulfill a kuleana would result in diminished mana" (Crabbe, Fox, and Coleman 2017, 39). This could lead to imbalance between kānaka, ʻāina (land), and akua, which could manifest as a physical illness (Krauss 1993). An aliʻi who lost mana because of improper actions would lose the respect of the people and could even be killed.

Artifacts, possessions, and parts of the body could also be imbued with mana. To honor this, artifacts were treated with great care, and Native Hawaiians might protect their mana by burying or hiding discarded hair or nail clippings, the umbilical cord from a baby's birth, or the bones of the dead (Crabbe, Fox, and Coleman 2017).

Native Hawaiians also believed that there was mana in language, particularly spoken language. Before the introduction of the written Hawaiian language, Kānaka chanted an oral record of history. "That oral record was our database," says Kamanaʻo. "Dependent on oral communication, Hawaiians developed high intelligence. Our brains had to have a large capacity to learn, recite, teach, and add to these long chants that documented our history."

In preparing the book *Mana Lāhui Kānaka,* the research team led by Dr. Kealoha Fox and facilitators Dr. Aukahi Austin and Kīhei Nahale-a interviewed Native Hawaiians about mana through focus groups. Participants spoke to the importance of collective mana to building lāhui (the Hawaiian nation) and contributing Hawaiian thought and mana in Oceania. One kupuna shared,

> It's [through] that collective power of the collective pule of the unification of our collective spirit and our collective mana that we were able to accomplish what we did. . . . What are the main things that we agree on? This is our ʻāina. We belong here. We're born out of these lands . . . we have the same moʻokūʻauhau, regardless of what moʻokūʻauhau you have. We all come from Hāloa. We all agree on those things. That's where we start, and that's how we build our nation. And for those places where we disagree, then leave it aside. We don't have to agree on everything right now. That's the way I think, and that's why I think if we could all agree on the larger issues, it's going to be so easy to build that Lāhui. Just take the bigger issues and leave the manini things aside. You know, you kūkākūkā about those manini things at another time, but on the big issues, what we agree on, this is where we start. That's our first kuleana. (Crabbe, Fox, and Coleman 2017, 208–209)

The Importance of Teachers

Kamanaʻo had many kumu who were significant mentors and role models. These included kumu Hokulani Holt-Padilla, Auntie Abbie Napeahi, Auntie Malia Kawaihoʻouluohāʻao Craver, Earl Kawaʻa, Richard Likeke Paglinawan, Billy Kahalepuna Richards, Gordon ʻUmi Kai, and others. These individuals shared their knowledge and guided Kamanaʻo's acquisition of skill in the practices of ritual ceremony, hoʻoponopono, lua, and many other Hawaiian cultural practices. They also embodied living examples of Kānaka makua or enlightened, matured, and esteemed models of true Hawaiian character.

Kamanaʻo also remembers Dr. Kekuni Blaisdell as a significant mentor and role model. To Kamanaʻo, Dr. Blaisdell exemplified this ʻōlelo noʻeau:

ʻIKE NO I KA LĀ O KA ʻIKE; MANA NO I KA LĀ O KA MANA.

Know in the day of knowing, mana in the day of mana.

(PUKUI 1983, 131)

He understood both Western and Hawaiian knowledge. If someone talked against Hawaiians, he would ʻōlelo pāpā or verbally challenge this person right away in a manner that was respectful yet empowering as a kanaka [Native Hawaiian]. Kekuni was a warrior, a healer, a priest, and an advocate for our lāhui. But he also was an academic and a scholar. He had mana because he was so knowledgeable. He was one of the first to point out the negative effects of colonization on the health of our people. He understood the Western way, but he was able to contextualize it and use it for our lāhui.

All of Kamanaʻoʻs mentors, including his parents, granduncle, and kumu, would tell him to nānā, which means to closely observe. In learning to observe people, you look at their behavior and how they conduct themselves. You listen to what they are saying and then see if their behavior is consistent with what they are saying. If so, you can conclude that this is a person of integrity, that this person is pono, and this is a reflection of mana. Kamanaʻo believes that the philosophical concept of mana is core to the foundation of Hawaiian thinking and behavior, going back to the basic values and beliefs of the Kānaka ancestors: "Mana is reflected through our heritage as a great, proud, and dignified people who harnessed the energies of our universe to build a society in tune with the physical, celestial, and spiritual realms of our existence."

Kamanaʻo is happy to see a strong desire among members of the millennium generation to learn Hawaiian culture. But he believes that kumu are important to the preservation of Hawaiian knowledge. "The shocking thing is that many young people are learning about Hawaiian cultural practices through YouTube. I was pūʻiwa [shocked] when I heard of this," he says. Although he believes that YouTube and Google are acceptable avenues for an introduction to the culture, to truly learn and preserve the integrity of Hawaiian culture, individuals should study with an esteemed, recognized, acknowledged teacher who comes from a legitimate line of formidable pillars of their traditions. "We must uphold the standard of preserving our

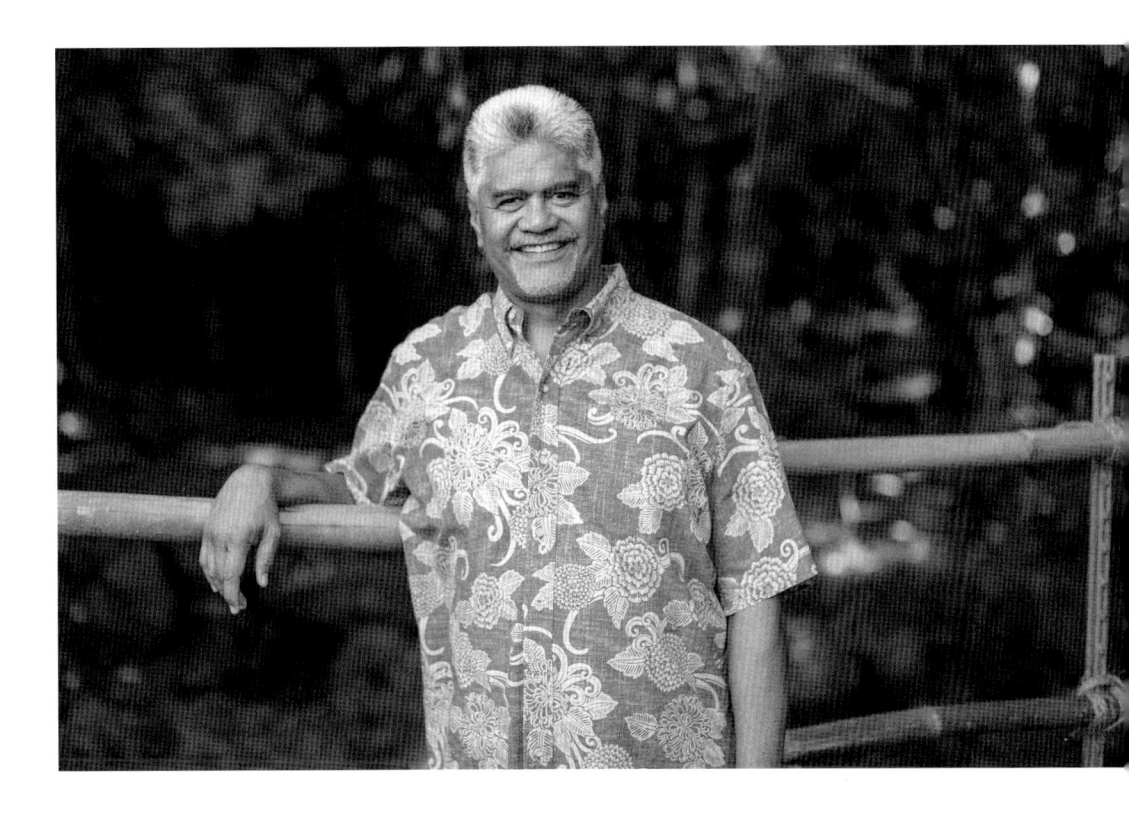

knowledge through the oral tradition and ways of cultural knowledge acquisition," he explains.

Teaching Others

Kamanaʻo is often asked to teach others about mana. Since the publication of the book *Mana Lāhui Kānaka,* he has been approached to develop a curriculum for teaching about mana. "I also was asked by two Māori clinical psychologists to engage with them in conversations about Indigenous psychology and what that might look like," he remembers.

Kamanaʻo recognizes that the Hawaiian way of learning is different from the academic way of learning. For example, through the ʻAha Kāne movement, Kamanaʻo taught Hawaiian language through ʻawa ceremony:

> I took different moʻolelo and we would kūkākūkā [discuss] the principal characters, themes, plots, cultural practices, and the secret

knowledge held within the web of folklores. When we learned an oli or mele, we talked about its meaning, what ʻike we were to glean from it, and how it is used in ceremony. They learned language through this way of teaching. As part of their graduation, they had to collectively recite and chant all of the different chants, in addition to making a traditional kapu imu (an oven for preparing food for a ceremony). They had to make their own kānoa (ʻawa bowls), apu (traditional coconut serving cups), strainers, malo, and kīhei (cloak).

As a medium for sharing sacred information, moʻolelo were believed to have mana (Crabbe, Fox, and Coleman 2017). The word "ʻōlelo" refers to speech or speaking. The word "moʻo" has important and interconnected meanings, including succession, series, to follow a course, a small fragment, and path (Pukui and Elbert 1986). Moʻolelo traditionally described the mana of sacred places, people, and historical events. Kamanaʻo is thankful to his granduncle Bob, who used moʻolelo to teach him the importance of moʻokūʻauhau, kuleana, and pono living. "Because in my day," he says, "we never heard of a psychiatrist or a psychologist. When my mom said 'go to your uncle,' that was old-school Hawaiian therapy."

Kamanaʻo also teaches about mana in his role as a parent. For example, he and his adolescent daughter talked about her response when she saw some of her classmates bully another classmate:

> When she talked to me about this, I asked her "What did you do?" She said, "I told them to stop it." Then I asked, "Why did you tell them to stop it?" She said, "Because they were picking on the other girl." Again I asked why, and she said, "Because I don't think that's fair." I said, "Good." But then the bullies started bullying my daughter, so I asked "What do you do?" She says, "I just ignore them." I said, "Good, you can ignore them, but you also need to protect your mana bubble. Don't let others penetrate your personal space physically, emotionally, and mentally. Tell them that they cannot be your friend if they do that, because that's not good behavior, and it's not what you believe." So I'm trying to teach her how to be pono, how to exercise her mana in an assertive way, but also how to defend it, protect it, and care for it.

Building Mana, Building Our Future

Kamanaʻo believes that today's Kānaka Maoli (Native Hawaiians) have to learn how to walk in both worlds. A good example of Hawaiians who do this well are the Mauna Kea kiaʻi (caretakers) (Hoʻomanawanui et al. 2019). Kamanaʻo believes they have great mana and are the epitome of what we strive to be. Many of the kiaʻi went through Pūnana Leo (Hawaiian immersion schools), so they know ʻōlelo Hawaiʻi and are steeped in the culture. He said, "They are walking the path, they have studied, and they are applying their knowledge for the good of our lāhui Hawaiʻi. They know their moʻokūʻauhau, they have confidence, they reflect mana as strength, they are intelligent, and they have good morals and integrity. We need to continue to create a contemporary understanding of mana and point out good examples. In this way, we can move forward and build on mana as a resilient, cultural strength and asset uniquely Hawaiian, uniquely Polynesian."

Could non-Hawaiians acquire mana? Kamanaʻo believes that this is possible. He points to Patience Bacon, a Japanese woman who was hānai by Mary Kawena Pukui in early childhood. Auntie Pat, as she was known in later life, learned the Hawaiian language and hula from Kumu Pukui. As an adult, Auntie Pat joined her mother as an employee of the Bishop Museum, translating Hawaiian language documents, nūpepa, and oral histories (Hurley 2021). Kamanaʻo reminds us that there are many non-Hawaiians who learn Hawaiian things. The question is, he says, "Do you have good character and integrity on how you carry out your life and the Hawaiian traditions you practice and live?"

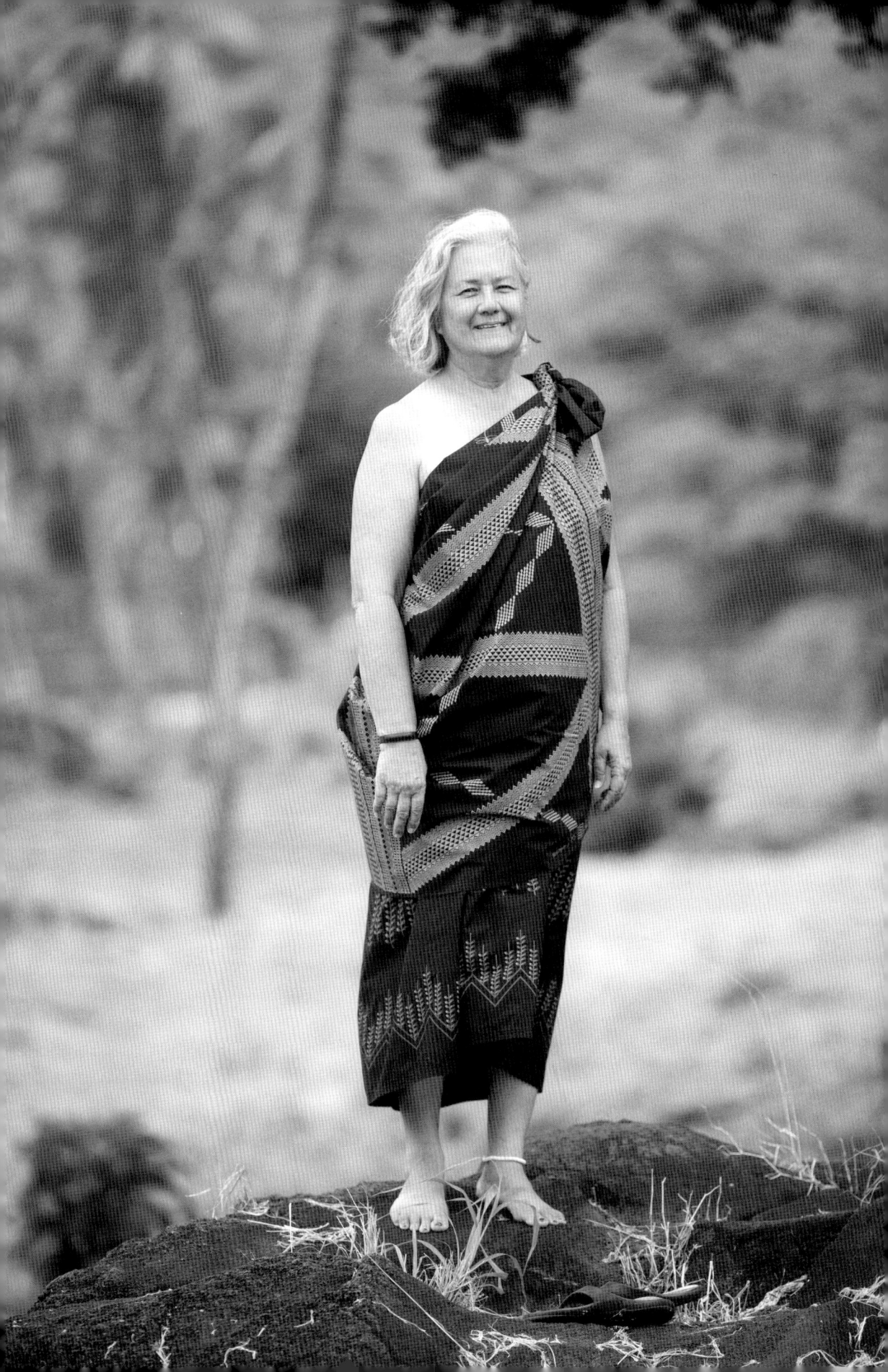

CHAPTER 3

Linda Kaleoʻokalani Paik

MĀLAMA KŪPUNA, MĀLAMA ʻĀINA

As gentle breezes rustle the leaves of the ʻulu (breadfruit) trees in the courtyard, people settle into their seats at the Bishop Memorial Chapel in the hills of Kapālama, Oʻahu. The chapel holds portraits of Ke Aliʻi Pauahi Bishop and Charles Reed Bishop, is adorned with kāhili (feather standards, symbol of royalty), and has as its center a solid sandalwood religious cross and an altar carved of coral. As people wait for the memorial of a beloved kupuna (elder) to start, the chapel is filled with the pure and melodious voice of Linda Kaleoʻokalani Paik, singing Ave Maria, a prayer set to music.

Voice of Advocacy

Kaleoʻokalani (Voice of the Heavens), known as Kaleo, was named by her grandaunt on her father's side. She feels that the name is prophetic, as she is trained in voice and enjoys singing. Generations of her family can be traced to South Kona. She notes that the speech of families of South Kona "is smoother, not so guttural, and seems more melodic and lyrical in a sense," which is appropriate for a gifted singer. During her lifetime, Kaleo has sung at family and community events, including birthday parties and holiday celebrations. Equally important, she has used her voice for advocating for Hawaiian causes that she defines as "mālama kūpuna, care for elders and ancestors and mālama ʻāina, care for the land."

Growing up in South Kona, Kaleo learned Hawaiian ways and practices from her family, and in particular from her father. One such complex practice related to helping loved ones in the passing from life to death. In her family, she was chosen to continue this practice. Her father felt it was important to understand and be able to help release a beloved from life to death. When he approached her, she admits she had to overcome her own self-doubts. It took her three years of thoughtful consideration before she felt ready to make the commitment to her family to learn a practice with such significant magnitude and gravity. She eventually expressed a "willingness to take on that great kuleana of helping family members in the passing from life to death."

Kaleo acknowledges that her way of dealing with the passage of life to death may be different from that of other people, but that the commonality is in the honoring of cultural values. For example, one value is knowing the importance of land for people and understanding that ancestral lands provide people with a sense of origin, place, and identity. Thus, it becomes vital that loved ones be buried in places that have meaning for their identity and their lives. She learned from her father not in the "school-style way" but by observing as she went with him to comfort families suffering grief and bereavement. She also feels that this kind of learning is supported by ancestral memory, in which Hawaiian ways are not lost, just forgotten until the right moment, when these practices are accessed anew. For Kaleo, there were moments when ways and sounds that were unfamiliar became familiar as ancestors placed new learning in her path.

Kaleo is resolute in stating that "the task is quite sacred, in all its dimensions." The practitioner must be selfless and committed to helping release and free the beloved from life to death. In being selfless, she feels that one's mana is 100 percent dedicated to the person to ease the transition from life to death. It is said that it is the job of the living family members to help others be at peace when it is their time to go, and that the ʻaumākua are waiting and will make the walk easy (Lee and Willis 1987).

As an example, Kaleo talked about the release of a very young child of a cousin who had a brain tumor and was in a coma in a hospital with little expectation for recovery. The parents of the young child were overwhelmed and distraught and knew they would have difficulties in releasing their child. Given Kaleo's role in the family, they asked her to be with their child. With compassion and resolute focus, Kaleo sat with the child. She prayed, listened, and received the spiritual message of confirmation to release. The child died soon thereafter. With Kaleo's support and guidance the parents found comfort in this difficult time.

The importance of release has been described as letting the spirit be free to leap "into eternity or Pō" (Pukui, Haertig, and Lee 1972, 131). There were cliffs on each island that were believed to be the leina-a-ke-akua, the place from which spirits leaped into eternity. The leap into eternity was viewed as permanent, except when there was a return to help the family in need: "If the god [with whom you are to dwell] wishes you to come back to help us in our time of need, come and then return to the presence of your god. You are on the trail on which there is no return, so let us seek the path ourselves when our time shall have come" (Handy and Pukui 1972, 149).

Mālama Kūpuna

Kaleo's experiences in supporting family members transition from life to death positioned her for advocacy of mālama kūpuna. For Kaleo, "kūpuna" refers to ancestors and living elders. "The inclusive term for deceased ancestors and living elders, kupuna, as representing the stock from which the ʻohana spring as off-shoots, was derived from the verb kupu ʻto grow' with the suffix ʻna' added" (Handy and Pukui 1972, 4). It is important to note that the reference to kūpuna is expanded to refer not only to elders but also to deceased ancestors who could have died as children, young adults, or older adults. Caring for our ancestors has also been known as mālama iwi (care for ancestral bones). Care and reverence for ancestral bones originates in the belief that "it was with the bones that the ʻuhane (spirit) remained identified" (Handy and Pukui 1972, 151), and that a person's "immortality was manifested in his/her bones" (Pukui, Haertig, and Lee 1972, 107). Thus the bones were sacred for the individual and the entire family. This sentiment is expressed in the following ʻōlelo noʻeau:

OLA NA IWI.

The bones live.

(PUKUI 1983, 272)

In her unique role in helping with the transition from life to death, Kaleo became knowledgeable about the Native American Graves Protection and Repatriation Act (NAGPRA 1990). This act addresses the return of human remains and cultural objects that have been excavated or discovered on federal or tribal lands to lineal descendants, tribes, or Native Hawaiian organizations. She also became involved with the Oʻahu Island Burial Council, a group associated with the State Historic Preservation Division of the Hawaiʻi State Department of Land and Natural Resources that focuses on the management of burial sites. Approximately 98 percent of the burial cases handled by the division relate to Hawaiian skeletal remains, and since 1991, about three thousand sets of Hawaiian skeletal remains have been reinterred (Hawaiʻi State DLNR n.d.). The interpretation of human and Indigenous rights and the return of remains and objects can be highly controversial and contested (NAGPRA 1990), and it is important that Hawaiians are involved in cultural practices that provide for the respectful care of ancestral remains. In 2007, Kaleo and other commissioners of the Oʻahu Island Burial Council advocated for the release of displaced iwi (bones) on a construction site on Keʻeaumoku Street. The remains of Hawaiian kūpuna had been in boxes on the construction site since 2005, and as Kaleo stated, "reburial is a priority. Having kūpuna in boxes underneath a parking ramp is not the ideal situation in any religion, any human sentiment" (Pang 2007). The remains on this site were eventually reinterred following the collaborative efforts of many people and organizations.

Attention to the disturbance of ancestral remains and reburial are increasingly important as more discoveries are being made. Burial sites are often accidentally disturbed either by nature (surf or erosion) or by human activity through excavation (Hawaiʻi State DLNR n.d.). Kaleo states that burial sites varied by region, and could be in the ground, in the sand, or in caves. With ancestral iwi that have been repatriated, Kaleo affirms "that there is no difference if the bones are that of an adult or a child, as they are kūpuna since they have passed before us." She emphasizes that we must put them "back into a place of respect and understanding. And not just a physical space, but a spiritual space."

Kaleo states that her four requirements of kanu (burial) may differ from those of others. She follows the practice that she learned from her family, which was observed over the years. The first is a requirement "of being selfless in order that your thoughts and actions go with the deceased. Your being has to be 100 percent with the kūpuna without any ulterior motive or outside thoughts." Kaleo speaks about "infusing my energy, infusing our light, to help kūpuna pass through this process." In the case of repatriation, which may involve the ancestral remains of several kūpuna, Kaleo states that the second requirement is "to ask them for forgiveness, not because you have disturbed them, but because someone did," and we must apologize for that act. The third requirement is to select a burial site that is respectful of the kūpuna and to ask them to "please accept the reburial places we have given you." The fourth requirement is to let the kūpuna know that we "must ʻoki [cut] all ties with them so that the ʻeha [pain, injury] does not stay, and they are able to move on." The emphasis is on helping the kūpuna move on in their journey and having the freedom to do so.

In her experience with repatriation, Kaleo acknowledges that much of what is discovered today are bone fragments. These fragments have to be labeled, wrapped, and placed in a container for reburial. While in the old days, kapa (traditional Hawaiian cloth) might have been used to wrap the bones, Kaleo suggests that today it is acceptable to "place the bones lovingly in a pūʻolo [container, bag], perhaps of muslin or linen, tie [it] with cordage, and put in a basket" ready for reburial.

While there may be many materials important for reburial, Kaleo identifies four in particular: water, paʻa kai (salt), ʻōlena (turmeric), and limu kala (seaweed). To ensure the sanctity of the process, her preference is to be able to grow the materials for one's use or gather the materials oneself from special places. But if that is not possible, she acknowledges that one may accept the materials from a trusted family member or friend. For example, she explains that one may grow the ʻōlena and gather the limu kala and then prepare them appropriately for reburial. But one can also accept the limu kala gathered by someone else. Water may be more difficult to obtain, as you "try to get the wai and the kai [salt water, ocean] from where the kūpuna are from." If that is not possible, she reminds us to use what is at hand—the ocean for the procurement of salt water, and bottled water to symbolize fresh water. There are historical accounts of the importance of these materials for purification ceremonies.

The wai huikala, or water of purification, was always required in a kala (untie, freeing, release) ceremony. It consisted of seawater, and if that was unobtainable, of fresh water with a little salt dropped into it. A pinch of ʻōlena root might be added if there was any at hand (Handy and Pukui 1972, 145).

Salt water has been recognized as a cleansing agent by Hawaiians from ancient times. Turmeric, which the Hawaiians call ʻōlena, has the power of defying evil (Gutmanis 1991, 8).

Limu kala, in a dish filled with seawater that also contained turmeric, was used for purification (Malo 1951, 97).

Kaleo places these ingredients into a bowl and uses the mixture for purification. While these ingredients are important in purification, Kaleo emphasizes that they have no spiritual power as separate ingredients. She states that "it is the practitioner who must make use of these ingredients and infuse energy into the bowl, reflecting a selflessness and pureness."

Kaleoʻs voice of advocacy for repatriation and interment is expressed in her poetry. She composed a tribute to kūpuna who were removed from their resting place and subsequently hidden in another place during construction at Kunia, Oʻahu. The poem speaks to the pain of desecration, the steadfastness of kiaʻi, the plea for balance, and the love of our kūpuna and ʻāina. An excerpt is shared here:

> *Upheaval of earth seen from a distance*
> *Cloud rising from the movement of the aina*
> *Clawing and digging, replacing what was*
> *Dissipating the energy into nothingness.*
> *The tears do not come, the pain is too deep.*
> *In solemn silence the kiai stand in vigil.*
> *Their hearts slowed to replace anxiety*
> *Their minds cleared to replace emotion.*
> *Action inevitable, though damage done*
> *The love of kupuna and aina above all else*
> *Drives the just into a course hard chosen*
> *The scale heavily weighted in loss.*
> *Prayers as spears thrown into the darkness*
> *Shattering ignorance into enlightenment*
> *These weapons of choice, intentional and sure*
> *Will bring balance once more to this aina.*
>
> (PAIK 2013, "KUNIA")

Mālama ʻĀina

For Kaleo, her care and her reverence for our ancestors easily translate into her advocacy for special places in Hawaiʻi. For many Hawaiians the intricate relationships of people, land, and the spiritual realm provide a perspective that guides beliefs, values, and ways. Kaleo acknowledges that the land plays a central role in the health and well-being of Native Hawaiians. Resources of the land—stones, water, and plants—are used for healing and for nourishment. She states that "in taking care of the land, Native Hawaiians provide for our own health." The following ʻōlelo noʻeau reflects the importance of people's careful stewardship of the land in feeding and nourishing its people:

HE ALIʻI KA ʻĀINA; HE KAUWĀ KE KANAKA.

The land is a chief; man is its servant.

(PUKUI 1983, 62)

In daily activities, Kaleo feels that the bond of people with the land is in knowing when to fish, plant, and harvest according to the ever-changing weather and seasons. She believes that the land has provided for generations of Native Hawaiians, and will hopefully provide for those yet to come.

With a commitment to mālama ʻāina, Kaleo has worked as a cultural educator and advisor to people and communities dedicated to protecting and preserving the land. For example, she worked as part of a larger community group to preserve a wahi pana in Maunalua, Oʻahu. This group involved many community volunteers and organizations, including the Livable Hawaiʻi Kai Hui and the Trust for Public Land. Together, they advocated for the preservation of the wahi pana of Hāwea heiau and the adjoining Keawāwa wetland in Maunalua. This is a historic site recognized for its precontact existence, with numerous petroglyphs, an ancient ulu niu (coconut grove), many ancient rock formations thought to be house structures, agricultural terraces, burial sites, and Hāwea heiau. It is believed that the canoe of the Tahitian voyager Laʻamaikahiki landed here with a pahu (drum) that was used ceremonially at the royal birthing grounds of Kūkaniloko at the center of Oʻahu (Livable Hawaiʻi Kai Hui n.d.; Trust for Public Land n.d.).

After years of neglect, in 2009, the site was threatened with destruction because of the proposed construction of a parking lot and public park. The community intervened to stop the construction. As part of an organized and peaceful protest, a "drumming" occurred at the site to call attention to the loss and imminent destruction of the sacred land. Supporters came to the drumming ceremony and those without drums were told to tap their chests over their hearts (Cataluna 2019). The successful outcome was the negotiated purchase of the approximately five-acre site of the Hāwea heiau complex to protect it in perpetuity (Cataluna 2019).

Since that time, Kaleo has worked with other advocates and the broader community in the cleaning, restoration, and preservation of the Hāwea heiau complex. Many have contributed, but there is a continual call for volunteers to help with land and cultural stewardship. Kaleo is known to direct people to areas where weeds must be pulled and toils side by side with them in this backbreaking work. In her role as cultural educator, she has taught visitors about the property's cultural and natural resources.

A culturally unique event occurred with the gift to the Hāwea heiau complex of a pahu made from a 112-foot-tall niu (coconut) tree from the grove of this sacred area. The tree was the tallest recorded niu in the state, but in 2014, high winds toppled her crown, and she started to decay. With careful stewardship and intense labor, Kaleo says that friends were able to bring the tree down without damaging any surrounding archaeological structures. The niu tree was sectioned off into smaller pieces, and kumu hula (teacher of hula) Brad Cooper took several months to craft a gift of a pahu from this magnificent niu. The cutaway designs in the pahu represent the hull of the canoe from Laʻamaikahiki. In 2015, with chanting rituals and a traditional ʻawa ceremony, the pahu was given as a gift, symbolizing respect for ancestral ways. Kaleo said, "There are no words that can competently express what it means to complete this process and achieve the dream we shared all those years ago." In 2019, the movement to preserve this sacred heiau reached the ten-year mark, and community members celebrated these ancestral lands (Cataluna 2019).

Kaleo's expression through poetry reflects her deep aloha for Hāwea. Her efforts of mālama ʻāina are rooted in spirituality, and she recognizes that our prayers are "less about asking Ke Akua [Christian God] for what we want, and more about asking Ke Akua for what we should do and the pathway to do it." In a poem, she wrote about the years of neglect of the land and the spirit of Hāwea calling out to those who are committed to the preservation of legendary places and cultural ways.

The drums of Hawea are silenced,
Years of neglect caused its demise.
A once prominent wahi pana,
Reduced to rubble and ruin,
Scarred pohaku caused by ignorance,
Left in a pile of disgrace.
A pohaku canvas paints
The history of those long gone.
Sacred aina used, as was pono,
To build a kauhale, heiau,
Sacred enclosures for our people,
To come and pay respect.
The essence of the spirit within Hawea
Calls out to be heard.
The vibration echoing the pulse
Of those who have made a stand.
For the sanctity of the Pahu,
The drum to unite us all.

(PAIK 2009, "HAWEA")

Calling for Pureness and Light

Kaleo has used her voice to express a commitment to culture through melodious song, riveting poetry, and words commanding cultural stewardship and preservation. As she looks at her life, she notes that her original reluctance to carry on the family responsibility for helping loved ones with the passage from life to death is replaced today with joy in knowing that she can help family members and others with the transition. She also experiences a quiet elation in honoring the kuleana of caring for our ancestors through repatriation and reburial and caring for sacred lands. In much the same way that she was chosen by her father to learn family practices as the punahele (special child), her granddaughter has been chosen as the next person in her family to

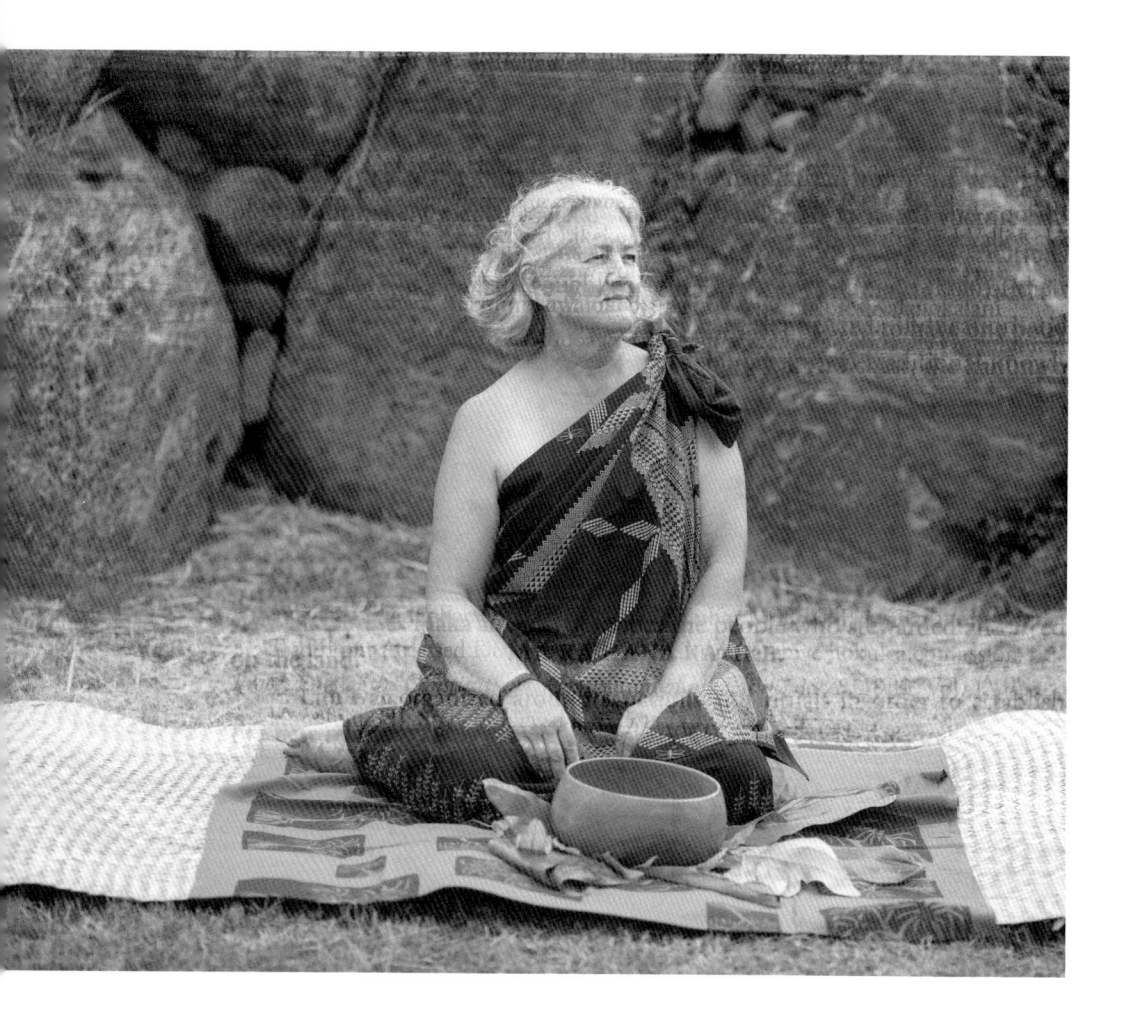

learn these practices. Kaleo says, "She is my punahele, and she is the one who will follow in my footsteps and who I will train."

Her message for students at the university interested in cultural advocacy for social justice and health equity is to first and foremost seek the pureness that lies deep within themselves. It is this pureness that will help them cultivate the compassion for helping others through challenging moments in life. She willingly teaches people about the materials required for reburial or instructs and models the behavior requisite for ceremonial protocol, but she is quick to emphasize the importance of being selfless and fully dedicated to people and places. Knowledge and skills, inherited and learned, are important, but they are secondary to the character and conduct of the practitioner.

Kaleo reiterates that it is the spiritual essence of the practitioner that is of paramount importance in mālama kūpuna and mālama ʻāina. This essence is reflected in the qualities of pureness and light as demonstrated through selfless behavior. Kaleo notes the beautiful family story of Pali Lee and Koko Willis in the *Tales from the Night Rainbow* (1987), which speaks about perfect light and the endless opportunities to grow that light:

> Each child born has at birth, a Bowl of perfect Light. If he tends his Light it will grow in strength, and he can do all things—swim with the shark, fly with the birds, know and understand all things. If, however, he becomes envious or jealous[,] he drops a stone into his Bowl of Light and some of the Light goes out. Light and the stone cannot hold the same space. If he continues to put stones in the Bowl of Light, the Light will go out and he will become a stone. If at any time he tires of being a stone, all he needs to do is turn the bowl upside down and the stones will fall away and the Light will grow once more. (Lee and Willis 1987, 19)

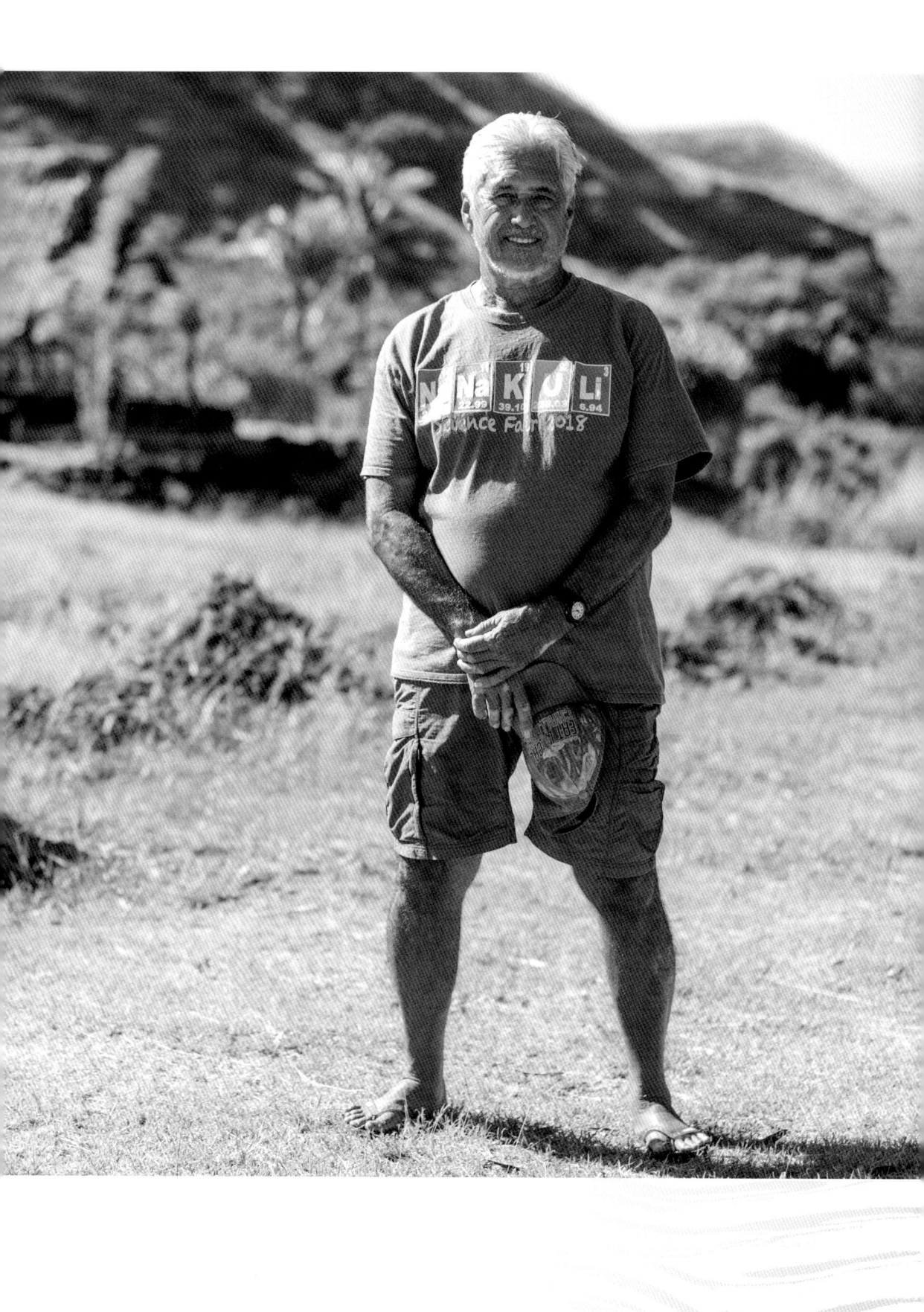

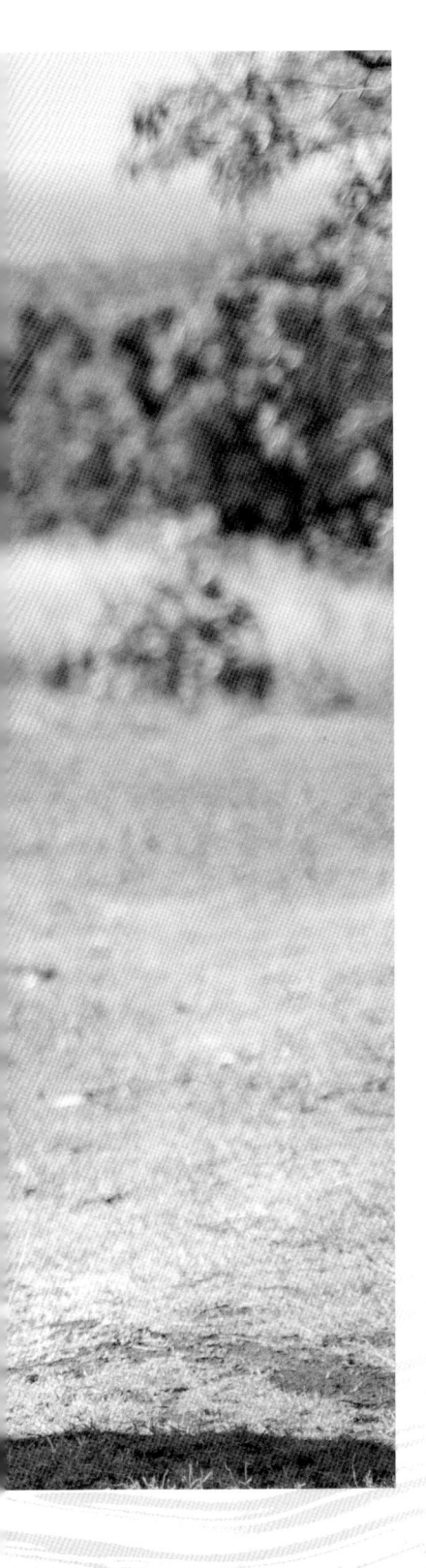

CHAPTER 4

Eric Michael Enos

'ĀINA MOMONA

Eric Enos has been reconnecting community with 'āina for more than forty years, and Ka'ala Farm in Wai'anae is an integral part of the movement to build healthy watersheds that sustain communities. Ka'ala Farm is an example of how the land can be returned to 'āina momona. "Momona" is a Hawaiian word that can mean fat, fertile, plump, rounded, or sweet (Pukui and Elbert 1986). In combination with the word "'āina," the phrase evokes "fertile, fruitful land and ocean," a land that is abundant and sustaining of human life and well-being. "To rebuild 'āina momona, we all have the kuleana and privilege to mālama [care for] this place," says Eric. An appropriate 'ōlelo no'eau is:

NA KE KANAKA MAHI'AI KA IMU Ō NUI.

*The well-filled imu (oven) belongs to
the man who tills the soil.*

(PUKUI 1983, 245)

Eric advocates for and strives to create 'āina momona in his and other communities. He explains, "The poor health of Native people everywhere is linked to the destruction of the Native environment and Native systems. Reconnecting communities with the 'āina and creating 'āina momona can help them to heal and thrive. Food health, land health, watershed health . . . these can help us huli (turn over) this poor-health trap with action."

Growing Up with an Appreciation for the 'Āina

Eric was born in Kalihi, but the family moved to the Mākaha area of the Wai'anae Coast of O'ahu when Eric was a baby. This area is a high-density Native Hawaiian community. Eric's mother was from the Ho'omanawanui 'ohana in the Kona area on the island of Hawai'i, and his father, who was part Portuguese, Japanese, and Hawaiian, was from Kaua'i. When Eric's parents moved to the Mākaha area, much of the land was recovering from the closure of the sugar plantation, with wild sugarcane still growing on the land and just a few houses. Eric's father was a machinist at Pearl Harbor, and his parents built their own home, even mixing their own cement and doing their own wiring and plumbing. The family also had a flower garden, and grew carnations, pīkake (jasmine), and pakalana (Chinese violet) for lei (garland) making. "My dad set up a whole automated bench misting system for propagation of plant cutting. So I learned farming from him, and patience from my mom in sewing lei," remembers Eric.

When Eric was growing up, the Wai'anae Coast looked much different than it does today. There were sand dunes on the beach, and then there were lowlands that were prone to flooding. Eric also remembers the whole area being filled with large mango trees. The area was thick and green, and there were plenty of freshwater springs. The river that fed Wai'anae town used to go by the heiau at Pu'ukāhea near Pōka'ī Bay. This area is rich in cultural history and is associated with the prophet Ka'opulupulu, who was renowned for his oracles in the late 1700s (Nakuina 1904). It also was part of the communication system with heiau on other points on the ridge and in the valley or by the shore along the Leeward coast. Before the establishment of the sugar plantations, Native Hawaiians could paddle their canoes and land at the base of the pu'u (hill) on which the Pu'ukāhea heiau was built.

But when the plantations came, much of the land was cemented and bulldozed. Parts of the water system became toxic because of runoff from the dairies and pesticides, and then a sewage outfall was built from Malaea to the ocean. "As most conquerors who demonstrate their power by desecrating religious site[s], one of the first sugar plantation managers who moved to the area tore down the heiau at Puʻukahea and built his mansion right on the site," says Eric.

Connections of Art, Activism, and ʻĀina

Eric attended the Kamehameha Schools and the University of Hawaiʻi at Mānoa (UHM) in the 1960s. At UHM, he studied art and art education. There were very few Native Hawaiian students at UHM then, and Eric remembers being asked if he was from India. While at UHM, he did his student teaching at Waiʻanae High School. He met some outstanding teachers who got involved in the community and got to know the children and their families. He admired them and tried to learn what he could. But he also met teachers who were very vocal about their dislike of the community and its people. Many of these teachers were biding their time in Waiʻanae, waiting for transfers to schools in more upscale communities. "They didn't like the kids, and so the kids didn't like them . . . it was circular," says Eric.

After Eric finished his student teaching, he volunteered at Nānākuli Park, where many young Native Hawaiians were hanging out, and he got them involved in art. Eric's approach to art and his approach to working with youth were influenced by the turmoil and movements of the 1960s and 1970s. He recalls, "There were struggles around Vietnam, Black Power, the Chicano and American Indian movements, the Hawaiian Renaissance, Kahoʻolawe, *Hōkūleʻa,* Chinatown evictions, Kalama Valley, and Waiāhole Valley. Many artists were involved in these movements, deciding that art was a vehicle to both free our minds and express social conditions. This was art for social change, the art of the streets."

Eric was most interested in social activism art in line with the muralist Diego Rivera, who painted about the working people of Mexico, and Pablo Picasso, who painted *Guernica,* which depicted the horrors of the civil war in Spain in the 1930s. He also studied and admired the US government's efforts in the 1930s to support art and artists during the Depression through programs such as the Civilian Conservation Corps (Lampert 2013).

When Eric graduated from the university, he was hired as a counselor by the Waiʻanae Rap Center to continue his work with the park gang at Nānākuli Park. The Rap Center was funded in part by Model Cities, a component of president Lyndon Johnson's War on Poverty (Weber and Wallace

2018). The initiative's goals emphasized comprehensive planning, involving not just rebuilding but also rehabilitation, social service delivery, and citizen participation.

Wai'anae has always been a rough place. Eric remembers, "The gangsters were running the kids, the kids ran in gangs themselves, and there was a lot of drinking at home. So we tried to offer the youth activities to try to point them in better directions." Besides doing art, Eric and the other counselors took the youth hunting and fishing. They organized programs to teach the youth about water safety and lifesaving. They were able to provide Aqua-Lung training so youth could master skills for jobs as divers, while the youth shared traditional ways to lay nets and clean fish that they had learned from their families. To support these activities, Eric and the other counselors learned about different nonprofits and funders and secured resources for the youth. They also helped the youth access job training programs so they could learn skills and earn money.

'Āina Momona: The Birth of Ka'ala Farm

In the late 1960s, the Wai'anae Rap Center received access to ninety-seven acres of state land that would later become Ka'ala Farm. Center administrators initially thought this land might be a place for youth clubs to go camping. "There was no identity of what this place was, and the land was overgrown and had been used as a dump. The stream was dry, and the place was a desert," remembers Eric. In the early 1970s, he and the Rap Center youth started cleaning the land by removing all the stolen cars that had been abandoned in the creek bed and along the road.

When the group started to hike up the valley toward the mountains, they saw well-constructed rock walls. They realized that these walls were the remains of a sophisticated irrigation system built by their precontact Hawaiian ancestors for the cultivation of taro and other plants to sustain life in the valley. They could see how the ancient water system brought water down from the mountain, directed it through the 'auwai (water channels), and spread it across the valley. "Although at the time the valley was a desert, we realized that, before colonization, the whole back of Wai'anae Valley was a poi bowl [fertile place for growing food]" says Eric.

From the mountain, they could see the practicality of the ahupua'a, a traditional land division that starts in the mountain and ends in the ocean, bounded by the valley walls. Prior to Western contact, the five biological resource zones of the ahupuaʻa supported human settlement and community life. These included the wao nahele (upland forest zone), the wao kanaka (agricultural zone), the kahawai, the kahakai (coastal zone), and the kai. This vertical land division system allowed communities to access a maximum of biodiversity and to honor the interactive influences of the five zones (Malo 1951; Mueller-Dombois 2007). Wai comes from the mauna (mountain, watershed) and is essential to support plant and animal life.

The group also saw how the plantations had diverted the water and starved out or evicted the Native Hawaiians living in the valley. This realization gave deep meaning to an ʻōlelo noʻeau that describes what happens when water is taken away from the land:

PŪʻALI KALO I KA WAI ʻOLE.

Taro, for lack of water, grows misshapen.

(PUKUI 1983, 296)

In restoring the land, Eric and the youth cleared the haole koa (invasive species from the mimosoid tree family) and restored the loʻi. They cultivated the plants that were important to the Indigenous peoples of the valley, including taro, lau hala (pandanus leaf), and wauke (paper mulberry tree). Kaʻala Farm became a nonprofit organization in 1976, was incorporated in 1983, and received tax-exempt status in 1988. Around the same time, the land was turned over to Hawaiian Homelands, with a licensed agreement between the entities. Kaʻala Farm's mission became reclaiming and preserving the living culture of the poʻe kahiko (people of old) in order to strengthen the kinship relationships between the ʻāina and all forms of life necessary to sustain the balance of life on these venerable lands.

Kaʻala Farm as Kīpuka

Eric also refers to Kaʻala as a kīpuka. Eric describes "kīpuka" as an area of land ranging from several square meters to several square kilometers that supports plants and wildlife but is completely surrounded by lava. "Pele was the natural kīpuka builder. The lava surrounds the old growth, and the old growth becomes the nursery for the new growth" says Eric. "Places like Kaʻala Farm are kīpuka or puʻuhonua (places of refuge), surrounded by man's destruction of the environment. We reflect a community vision for cultural kīpuka and land-based kīpuka, places where our ancestral knowledge lives on through youth, where thriving ahupuaʻa are living examples of healthy, maintained watersheds, and where our Hawaiian traditions are carried forth in a way that strengthens our people and our communities."

To promote these messages, Kaʻala Farm has an educational center, offers community sessions and workdays, and runs an internship program. It also serves as an alternative school for youth, principally from the Waiʻanae Coast but also from Kapolei and other communities. The school uses a place-based learning approach, meaning that the curriculum is linked to the Waiʻanae Valley. Children and youth learn by engaging all their senses—sight, hearing, touch, taste, smell—and converting these sensations into a passion to understand and apply their knowledge to their communities. Working together, the teachers at Waiʻanae High School and the staff at Kaʻala Farm developed science, math, and advocacy projects for the youth. For example, over a series of years, the youth completed research on the water situation in the valley. They wrote and testified in support of a resolution at the national convention of the Association of Hawaiian Civic Clubs to protect the watershed, the forest, and traditional water uses in Hawaiian communities. In doing this, they learned how to estimate the water recharge of the loʻi and how to develop and present a persuasive argument. This approach to learning was very successful. "When these young people returned to school to take the exams, 100 percent passed, which meant they did better than the school as a whole. It's an amazing transformation when you see kids get interested in learning," says Eric.

Eric's commitment to establishing Kaʻala Farm as kīpuka and providing place-based education steeped in Hawaiian culture was based on his life experiences and the numerous mentors he had as an adult. While he may have gained an appreciation for the ʻāina from his parents during his formative years, Eric does not remember receiving any formal education in Hawaiian culture. "We didn't speak Hawaiian in my house, and exposure to Hawaiian culture at Kamehameha School was primarily limited to extracurricular activities," he says. His experiences and relationships with mentors provided his educational base. These mentors were diverse, but all prioritized cultural learning and ʻāina momona. For example, Eric and his youth group went to visit Lyon Arboretum in Mānoa. There, they met Donald Anderson, a researcher at the arboretum, who had a large collection of kalo (taro).

"Don Anderson was one-eighth Hawaiian, and he was so excited to see Hawaiian kids," remembers Eric. Don visited Kaʻala Farm and gave the group advice on which varieties of kalo to grow in which environments, and he explained the history and importance of each variety. Eric also met Beatrice Krauss, who wrote extensively about Hawaiian plants and lāʻau lapaʻau (Krauss 1993), and he started cultivating these as well.

Another plant that grew well at Kaʻala Farm was wauke. At first, Eric and the youth did not understand how to use the wauke to make kapa. But then they found a class on kapa making offered at the Hawaiʻi Nature Center in Makiki. "In the mid-1980s, we learned about kapa making from Auntie Alice and Dalani Tanahy Kauihou, and kapa making then became a regular activity of Kaʻala Farm," remembers Eric.

Other mentors included Uncle Walter Paulo and Uncle Eddie Kaʻanana, both from Miloliʻi on the island of Hawaiʻi, who were fishing for ʻopelu (mackerel scad) in the traditional Hawaiian way on Sand Island on Oʻahu. Both of these men were designated as living treasures of Hawaiʻi in 2006 for their contributions to preserving Hawaiian culture (Roig 2006). With Eric, they developed and obtained funding for their ʻOpelu Project, through which the youth learned to build and fish from ʻopelu fishing canoes. The group also used these canoes to teach the youth sailing, and they sailed around the island of Oʻahu. Never one to miss an opportunity for place-based learning, Eric worked with Linda Gallano, the Hawaiian studies teacher at Waiʻanae High School, to incorporate lessons on science into the project.

In addition to facilitating lessons in traditional fishing practices, Eric worked with the youth to learn hale (house) building, traditional farming, and making pōhaku ʻulumaika (stones used in a Hawaiian traditional game), papa kuʻi ʻai (board on which poi is pounded), and pōhaku kuʻi ʻai (poi pounder). They were informed by the books written by Te Rangi Hiroa, the first Western-trained anthropologist of Polynesian (Māori) ancestry (Thompson 2019). Also known as Sir Peter Buck, Te Rangi Hiroa was a world-renowned expert in Polynesian crafts and the director of the Bishop Museum from 1936 to 1951. His books, later compiled into a single volume, *Arts and Crafts of Hawaii,* provided rich descriptions of Hawaiian traditional objects, their uses, and their methods of construction (Hiroa 1957). The books also were used to identify Hawaiian artifacts found on Kaʻala Farm as the land was cleared. "So we did our research," Eric said. "We were working with the Bishop Museum, we were working with forestry, we were

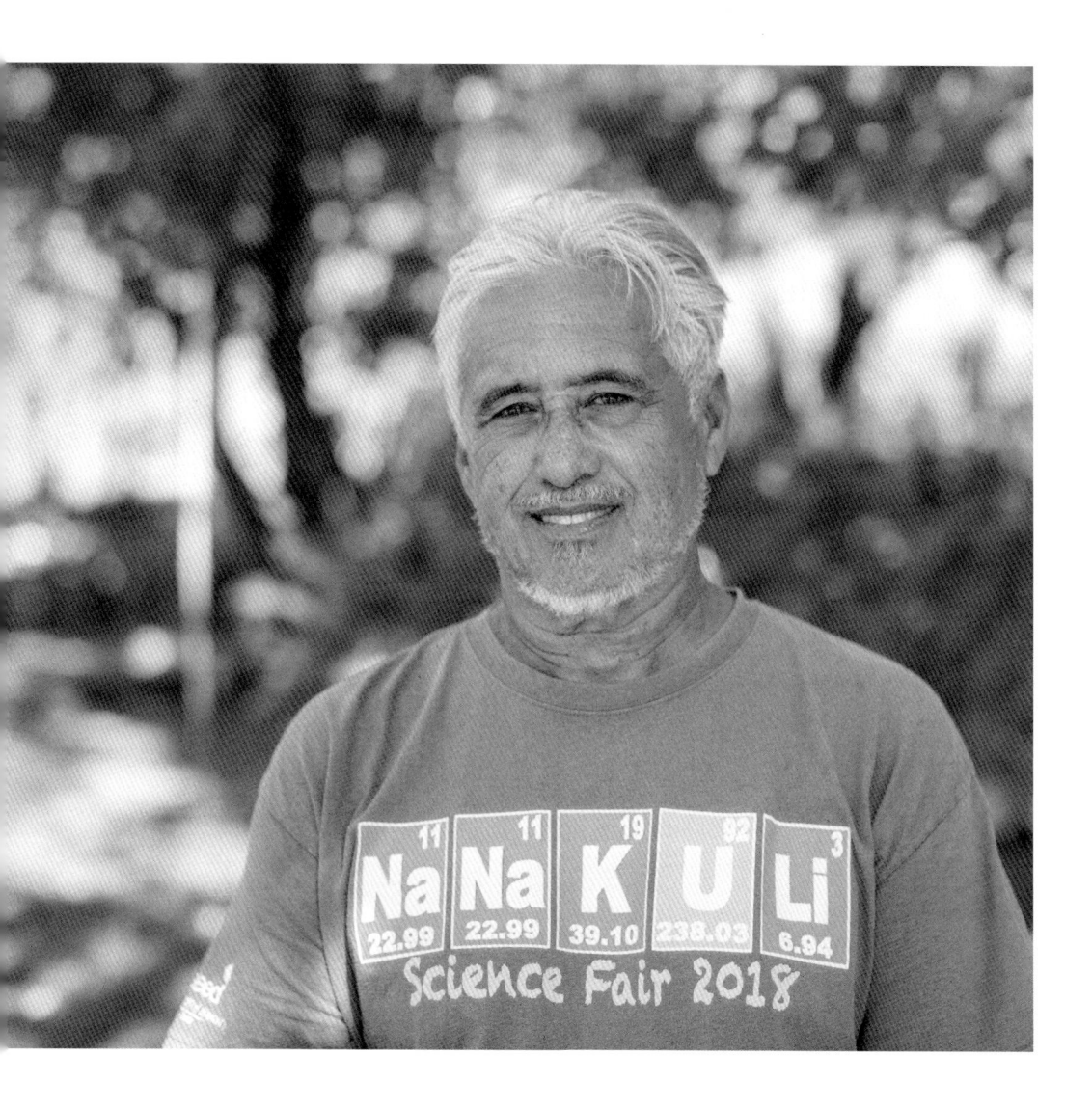

networking with all of these agencies, we sought grants for new projects for the kids, and many helped us."

Much of the knowledge accumulated by Ka'ala Farm over the years is included in a book, *From Then to Now: A Manual for Doing Things Hawaiian Style* (Ka'ala Farm 'Ohana 1996). The book was based on traditional Hawaiian knowledge from kūpuna (elders, ancestors) and other teachers who helped Eric, and included instructions on planting native species, preparing native foods, fishing, cleaning fish, making an imu (underground oven), and more.

"As we bring back the water to the valley, we need to be cognizant of our kuleana. We need to have guidelines and protocol to ensure the historical and cultural integrity of our work," says Eric.

Helping Others Build Kīpuka

Eric was involved in a number of other struggles to maintain Hawaiian land and culture, to build kīpuka, and to restore 'āina momona. In the 1970s, for example, Eric and other Rap Center counselors took their youth group to Waiāhole Valley. At that time, the state government had agreed to allow the building of seven hundred condo units in the valley. There were many kalo farmers living there, but they were on month-to-month leases, with no protection, and the city was planning to evict them to make way for development. Eric's group drove over from Wai'anae, bringing coolers filled with fish from the ocean. "At the time, we knew very little about kalo, but we heard there was a resistance, and we needed to find out what was going on. They welcomed us in, and we practiced nonviolent resistance with them." Later, the state purchased the land, and the evictions were forestalled (Nakata 1998).

In 1979, Eric brought his youth to help clear five acres of unused land in Mākaha that belonged to Sacred Hearts Church. This kīpuka became Hoa 'Āina O Mākaha, a farm and cultural learning center managed by Gigi Cocquio, a former Maryknoll priest. The Wai'anae Rap Center established an alternative school at Hoa 'Āina O Mākaha in connection with Ka'ala Farm, and for seven years they shared a tractor, which they would drive between the two farms.

In the 2000s, Eric also got his youth program participants involved in the restoration of Kū'ilioloa Heiau at Pōka'ī Bay. This heiau had been built by Lonokaeho, a legendary navigator, who brought some of the stones for the heiau from his home country, Tahiti. The heiau was surrounded on three sides by ocean and served as a school for navigation and a blessing site for voyages. The bay, Pōka'ī, was named for the navigator Pōka'ī, who is said to have brought coconut palm trees to Hawai'i, which provided both food and shelter for the early Hawaiian people.

Also in the 2000s, Aulani Wilhelm, an environmental activist, brought her brother Dean to Ka'ala Farm. They started talking about the negative effects of colonization and how Kānaka Maoli should take back the land, starting in their own backyards. Eric remembers,

Dean went back home, and he and his wife Michele found a place in Maunawili that had been an old rice field. It couldn't be developed because it was so wet, so they got it for a pretty good price. They built a tree house and started to restore the area. They planted kalo and started a poi business. This became Hoʻokuaʻāina. Today, they sell kalo and poi, sponsor community work days and internships, and work with kids. This is an example of how people can see our struggles to reclaim the ʻāina and the wai, and take what we're doing to build their own ʻāina momona in their own ahupuaʻa.

Advancing Social Justice and Health through ʻĀina Momona

Community farms, restoration projects, and place-based learning centers across the state of Hawaiʻi have drawn inspiration and know-how from Kaʻala Farm. Eric's dedication was recognized by a Hoʻokele Award from the Hawaiʻi Community Foundation in 2002, and as a "Planner Who Has Made a Difference" by the University of Hawaiʻi in 2006. But the struggle to build ʻāina momona continues. Eric extended this invitation at the ʻAha Kāne conference in 2012:

> Join us in a journey that never ends. We can be that generation that stood up, put aside our differences, and found common ground to build hope. Bring a gift to the circle, step out of your silo, and give our children hope and skills to build peaceful, healthy communities. Every one of you, in your moku, in your ahupuaʻa, there are places where there is māla, there is water, we have our rights, and we have our kuleana. From mauka to makai, from the ridge to the reef, it's all still here. This is what we mean by Kū Kiaʻi Mauna—stand up for the health of your ʻāina, the health of your mauna, and the health of your kai. You can help rebuild ʻāina momona. (Enos 2012)

Eric urges people to work together and to weave individual efforts into a basket of "net" works:

> One fisherman can catch a fish. But when the village gets together and everyone brings cordage and weaves a net that catches the whole school of fish, the whole village eats fish, and no one goes hungry.

The excess fish is salted, dried, and stored for future needs and bartered for goods and services. We manage our environment to guard when to fish, where to plant, and we distribute the natural resources wisely and sustainably. A healthy village has pono leadership that brings family leaders together and weaves resources into that healthy net. In this way, we can use the ʻāina momona movement to achieve health equity and social justice.

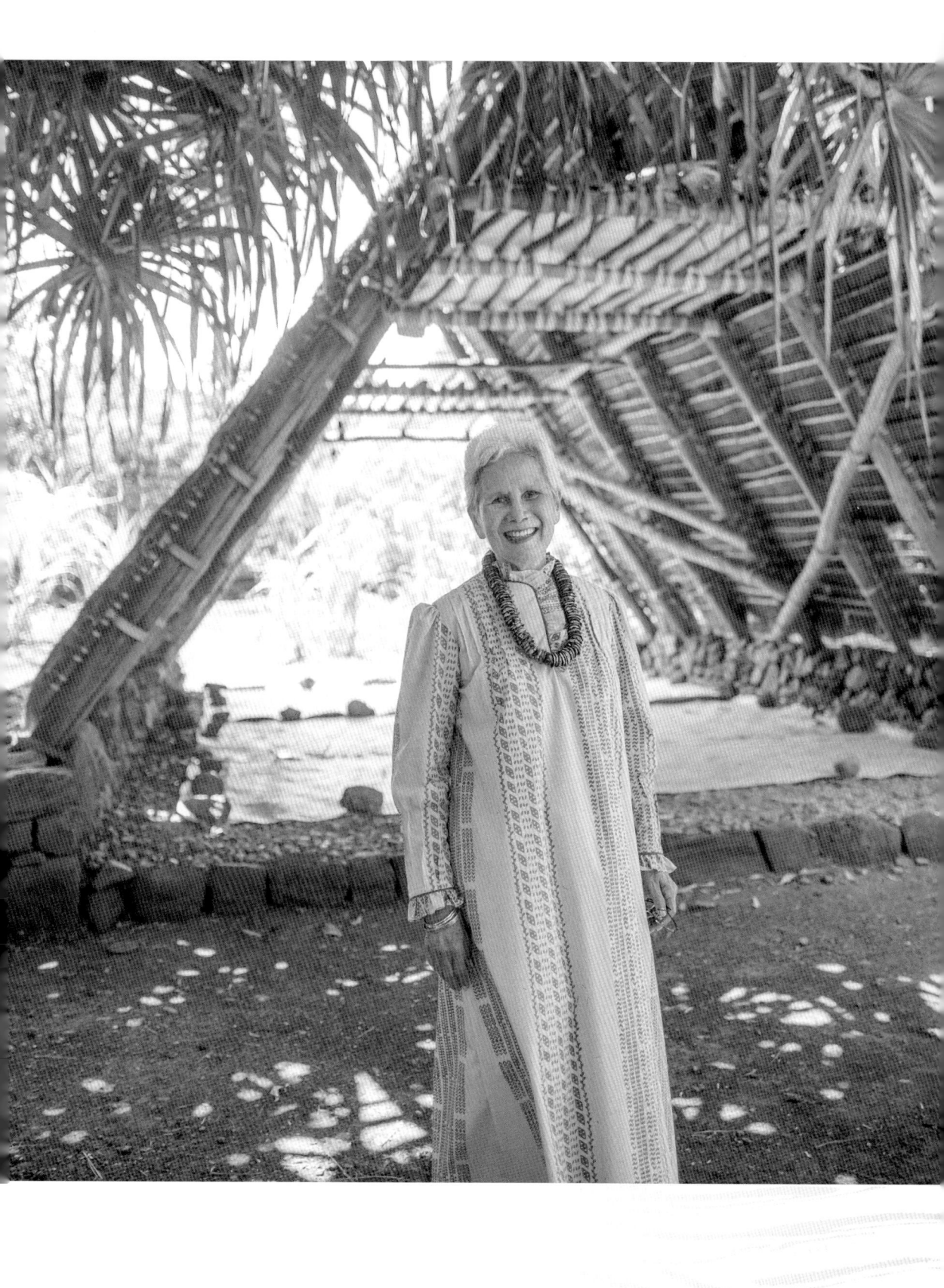

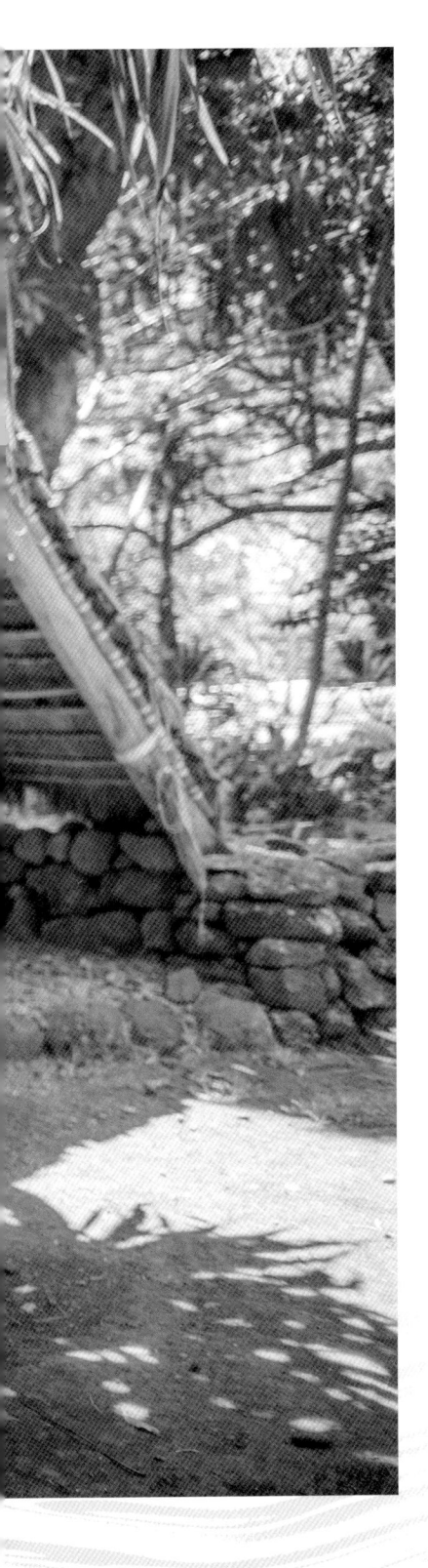

CHAPTER 5

Claire Kuʻuleilani Hughes

ʻAIAOLA

D r. Claire Kuʻuleilani Hughes has a fierce, lifelong commitment to improving our health by turning to traditional Hawaiian foods. Claire tells of how she chose this direction in childhood. Her mother, who guided Claire toward choosing a "purposeful life," frequently asked, "What do you want to be?" Suggestions that she become a teacher or librarian were rejected, always. Finally, in about the eighth grade, Claire was given a deadline for an answer. When confronted, her mind raced. She tried a joking response. Anger was clear on her mother's face as Claire struggled to provide a dutiful response. She recalled seeing a school newsletter article on dietetics and the importance of food, and while she was not totally clear on the education and training of a dietitian, she had an answer! She boldly told her mother, "I know exactly what I want to be. I want to be a registered dietitian."

An Early Calling

Decades later, Claire would recognize this as a hōʻailona (important sign and message from ancestors). The feeling that her ancestors were shaping her commitment to champion health by helping people to eat nutritious foods—'aiaola—became a central part of her life. Claire became the first Native Hawaiian registered dietitian in 1959, the first Native Hawaiian public health nutritionist in 1965, and the first Native Hawaiian branch chief of the Nutrition Branch of the State of Hawai'i Department of Health in 1992.

Like other children, Claire's first exposure to her life's priorities came from her family's lifestyle, which provided informal training on Hawaiian foods and practices. Claire was born on O'ahu, but grew up on a sugar plantation camp in Kekaha, Kaua'i, in the late 1930s, where there were clear lines of racial and ethnic segregation. Her father, who was Hawaiian-Welsh-English, was the plantation's engineer, and thus of the supervisory class, so, according to Claire, "the family lived in the haole camp." Her mother, who was Hawaiian-Scottish, had kahu hānai (adopted family) who raised her; they were Hawaiian, spoke only Hawaiian in their home, and fostered strong links with their Hawaiian ancestry. In Kekaha, the family formed friendships and spent time with other Hawaiians. It was during this formative time that Claire began learning about traditional Hawaiian foods, such as poi (pounded taro), a staple of the Hawaiian diet. Claire learned that reverence for the taro was based on its association with the Hawaiian gods Kāne and Lono. "Thus, poi was viewed as a sacred food as it was mixed and gently placed on the table last, and, after prayer, shared with everyone at the table, and covered between uses," says Claire.

Growing up, Claire learned that education would help her to achieve her goals in diet and nutrition. Her early education provided by her family was complemented by her formal Western education at Oregon State University (her father's alma mater) and at the University of Hawai'i at Mānoa, where she received a master's of science in public health and a doctorate in public health. Her doctoral studies focused on the traditional Hawaiian diet and its implications for culturally relevant promotion of health. In her studies, she assisted Drs. Kekuni Blaisdell and Emmett Aluli, and learned about the historical importance of Hawaiian foods in promoting health.

Claire recalls encounters with 'Ōlohe lua Charles William Lu'ukia Kaho Kemoku Kenn in which she asked him about the health of the first migrating Hawaiians to these islands. As is the style of teaching with many Hawaiian elders, he did not provide the answer but asked her, "What do you think?" Claire did not have an answer at that time, and made three more visits to 'Ōlohe (Master Teacher) Kenn before she gave a response that was acceptable. She said that the first Hawaiians "were the fittest and strongest.

The women were strong enough to assist during storms at sea, and during the long canoe journey. They were also able to help in the arduous work of establishing themselves in a new homeland." With an affirmative nod of his head, 'Ōlohe Kenn added that "they were the smartest ones, as well." 'Ōlohe Kenn and Claire agreed that in order to survive, these Hawaiians had to be most ingenious in farming, fishing, and building, and setting up a sustenance and sustainable society in their new island homeland.

Claire recalls historical written accounts denoting the health of Hawaiians through descriptions of their physical stature and activities. In an archaeological account of skeletal remains of Native Hawaiians in the 1700s, it was noted that "muscular bodies with very narrow hips were characteristic of these island people. The limb and hip bones showed extraordinary muscular development, in women as well as men. Indeed, all of their bones bespeak to the vigorous and strenuous outdoor existence of these people" (Snow 1974, 11).

This historical account is supported by other reports, and attribute physical health to diet and foods:

> The Natives of these islands [Hawaii] are, in general, above the middle size, and well made; they walk very gracefully, run nimbly, and are capable of bearing great fatigue. (Miller 1974, 167)

> We know that the Hawaiian people were splendid physical specimens and that their diet must have contained the elements necessary for health. (Handy et al. 1965, 95)

Historical Protocol for Food

As with many things in ancient Hawai'i, diet and food were governed by the kapu system, a code of conduct of standards and regulations. The kapu system has been described as the "keystone of the arch that supported the traditional culture of old Hawaii" (Handy 1931, 3). This system provided societal structure and functions that were based on religious beliefs and associated with mana. It was believed that the kapu system was established by the gods, and the ali'i, as descendants of the gods, were required to observe the kapu but were also holders of strong mana.

'Ai kapu was that system that specifically regulated food and eating practices. The establishment of 'ai kapu is attributed to Wākea. Claire states that "'ai" means "to eat, food," and "kapu" means "taboo." Claire notes that the main Hawaiian gods were associated with specific foods that were believed to be kinolau (forms taken by a supernatural body). Examples include:

* Kāne: taro, banana, ʻawa
* Kanaloa: banana, ʻawa
* Kū: breadfruit, coconut
* Lono: taro, certain fish
* Kamapuaʻa: sweet potato, pork, kukui

Claire states that the "'ai kapu was the strictest and most complex kapu[,] and everyone, from the aliʻi to the common man, had to follow ʻai kapu, absolutely." To deviate from these rules could result in death.

Under this cultural system, men ate in the mua (men's house), which was kapu to women, and women and children ate in the hale ʻāina (women's eating house), which was kapu to men. Claire notes that the tradition of restricted eating also meant that "every family man had to make two imu and cook food for men and women separately," and it was ultimately "the responsibility of the kūpuna for teaching the standards of ʻai kapu to their children."

The main food staple was the taro root, which must be well-cooked before being peeled and eaten or pounded and kneaded into poi. As starches, taro and poi have a high water and complex carbohydrate content and are good sources of many nutrients. Because taro represented the primordial man, only kāne (men) could cook the taro. And, customarily, the kāne prepared the poi and filled the calabashes for his wife, children, and other women in his family. Then the kāne did the same for himself and the other kāne in his family. "Poi was important for its nutrient value and strengthening the body, but it was also significant because of its spiritual value." Other foods in the traditional Hawaiian diet were sweet potatoes, bananas, coconuts, seaweed, fish, and chicken. Of all these foods, Claire is quick to note, "Poi is mana food."

Under the ʻai kapu system, there were certain foods that women were forbidden to eat. Some examples include most bananas, which were kinolau of the God Kanaloa; coconuts, which were kinolau of the God Kū; and the kumu fish, which was given as an offering in various rituals. The fact that women were forbidden to eat certain foods with high nutrient content bothered Claire, and so in her practice to always seek knowledge from her kūpuna, she asked the question of a Māori kahuna (expert), Hohepa, "Do the Māori have similar food restrictions for women?" When he answered affirmatively, she asked, "How is it that women could not eat kumu fish?" Kahuna Hohepa replied that the tradition "was intended as a protection for women. If a kumu fish was needed for a ceremony and none could be caught, the last person to eat the kumu fish could become the sacrifice. Women were protected because they give birth."

Claire notes that 2019 marked the 200th year since the abolishment of the kapu system by the powerful Queen Ka'ahumanu and her son, King Kamehameha II, in 1819. Their goal was to ensure the political authority of the Kamehameha line. They abolished the kapu system by having an open feast for men and women. By abolishing 'ai kapu, it was no longer necessary for men and women to eat in different houses, to have their foods prepared separately, or to have certain foods forbidden for consumption by women. Abolishing the kapu system and "displacing the arch" of traditional Hawaiian culture had many dramatic and dismantling effects on traditional Hawaiian culture. But Claire is quick to point out that, despite these significant losses, we can learn from the past about traditional practices. She states, "Our ancestors held important keys to their health that go largely unnoticed today. The traditional practices of lomilomi, family prayer, ho'oponopono, and timely treatment of illness with traditional herbs were vital keys to good health. Other equally important factors were the very high daily output of physical exercise necessary in farming, fishing, and canoe building and the wonderful traditional diet" (Hughes 2002, 5).

Traditional Hawaiian Foods to Improve Our Health and Wellness

For health advocates like Claire, there are many nutritious foods in the traditional Hawaiian diet, and Native Hawaiians and others can be encouraged to practice 'aiaola. Foods such as fresh fish, vegetables, and complex carbohydrates provide a solution to numerous health issues confronting Hawaiians today. Many Hawaiian communities experience a prevalence of obesity, resulting in disproportionately high rates of heart disease and diabetes when compared with other populations. Obesity may have a genetic basis, but it typically results from consuming more calories than are expended. There is a sadness in Claire's voice when she comments on our eating behaviors today: "There is a mindlessness in the way we eat today. We don't even chew our food. We eat with a chomp and chomp and swallow. We have forgotten the value of food and have no appreciation." More importantly, she states, "unlike our ancestors, we have no reverence for the foods we eat, and no appreciation of the relationship of gods and food." She thoughtfully contemplates that for many Hawaiians this behavior contributes to an emptiness and a search for solace that may derive from cultural loss as well as other factors.

Claire worked with numerous hoa aloha (friends) over four decades in establishing a pioneering dietary and nutritional intervention that would restore health. She credits Dr. Kekuni Blaisdell with the formulation of the nutritional composition table of the pre-Western Hawaiian diet and its comparison with a prudent adapted diet and typical American island diet (Fujita, Braun, and Hughes 2004). Illustrative highlights are identified in table 1. Claire was an avid reader of literature that supported her work with Dr. Blaisdell on the traditional Hawaiian diet. She identified the book *The Polynesian Family System in Kaʻū, Hawaiʻi* (Handy and Pukui 1972) as one of her best resources, and admitted to regarding it as a cultural "bible."

TABLE 1. COMPARISON OF PRE-WESTERN HAWAIIAN, PRUDENT ADAPTED, AND AMERICAN ISLAND DIETS

	Pre-Western Hawaiian	Prudent Adapted	American-Island
Carbohydrate (starch, fiber, sugar)	78 percent Kalo, ʻuala (sweet potato), ʻulu (breadfruit), hōʻiʻo (fern), limu (seaweed)	78 percent Taro, sweet potato, rice, fruits, seaweed, mango, guava	45 percent Rice, potatoes, noodles, fruits, vegetables
Protein	12 percent Iʻa (fish), pūpū (shells), ula (lobster), pāpaʻi (crab), moa (chicken)	12 percent Fish, seafood, chicken	15 percent Beef, pork, lamb, fish, chicken, legumes, eggs
Fat	10 percent Iʻa, moa, niu (coconut)	10 percent Fish, chicken, coconut	40 percent Beef, pork, lamb, sausage, nuts, butter, milk, eggs, cheeses

Table 1 was originally published in Fujita, Braun, and Hughes, "The Traditional Hawaiian Diet: A Review of the Literature," *Pacific Health Dialog* 11, no. 2 (2004): 250–259. Reprinted here with permission.

In 1987, using this formulation of foods and nutritional composition, Claire and Dr. Blaisdell worked with Dr. Emmett Aluli on Ho'okē 'Ai, also called the Moloka'i Diet Study, which tested the effect of the traditional Hawaiian diet on participants with high cholesterol levels. The goal was to see if changing the type of foods eaten, while holding calories constant, would lower participants' cholesterol, glucose, and blood pressure levels. Participants gathered at the Ho'olehua Recreation Center for their meals of traditional Hawaiian foods and participated in health monitoring activities and lessons. It required adjustment on the part of some participants, who were used to eating quickly and leaving the table, as they were reminded that it is a cultural practice to remain at the table until everyone is pau (done; to finish) eating. Claire chuckles and recalls that, on occasion, there would not be enough of certain Hawaiian foods, such as poi, on Moloka'i, so she would get an early morning phone call in Honolulu for help. "She would call different poi factories around Honolulu, pick up the poi during her lunch hour, drive to Honolulu Airport, and send it over to Moloka'i" (Wilcox 2011).

Claire and her colleagues believed that incorporating cultural values would improve health and contribute to cultural identity and self-esteem. The hope was that it would lend to instilling an appreciation for the sources and value of foods and culture. Values such as 'ohana, ho'omana (spirituality), and aloha 'āina (love for the land) linked food and nutrition to Hawaiian culture. The intervention was grounded in these values as participants ate together, started and ended meals with pule, and encouraged family members to join in educational sessions on cooking, the spiritual values of Hawaiian foods, and culture. In addition, study protocol included daily medical supervision and monitoring of outcomes, including cholesterol, glucose, triglycerides, blood pressure, and body weight. Body weight was held constant, so that changes in blood analyses could be attributed solely to dietary changes. Study results showed significant short-term improvements in these scores.

After the groundbreaking work on the Moloka'i Diet, Claire provided collaborative nutrition support to several people and groups. Foremost were Dr. Terry Shintani with the Wai'anae Diet Program in 1989, the State of Hawai'i Department of Health and the Native Hawaiian Health Care Systems throughout the islands in the 1990s, and Mr. Herbert Hoe with the 'Ai Pono Program in 1992. She also designed a nutrition and exercise program called Uli'eo Koa (warrior fitness, preparedness) in 2000. While the foundation for these programs was the traditional Hawaiian diet, modifications were made to ensure population reach and fit. For example, Dr. Shintani focused on weight loss and improved health, and included food choices of less-costly starches and vegetables from US sources. Mr. Hoe focused on health and participants who were very ill and their immediate family members. With Uliʻeo Koa, Claire focused on the traditional diet and introduced rigorous, daily physical activity with participants who were generally healthy and active in lua. A unique feature of Uliʻeo Koa was the assessment of spiritual and religious beliefs, with participants emphasizing Hawaiian spirituality and values, such as the belief in ancestral spirits.

While the short-term benefits in weight loss and health were demonstrated in all traditional diet programs, longer-term benefits were less clear. Like any weight loss or health program, once the intervention was completed, participants were challenged to sustain positive changes. Barriers included lack of access to traditional Hawaiian foods and other affordable food choices, limited physical exercise, and the lack of a support system among family, friends, and communities. In the course of her work, Claire is both fervent in her desire to help people through diet and nutrition, and fearful that she may fail with people who are highly vulnerable to disease and disability.

Looking Back, Moving Forward

Claire's destiny to care for Hawaiians through diet and nutrition was shaped by ancestors and started with her mother's query "What do you want to be?" As she finished telling us her story, she reminisced about her mother, Violet Kimokeo Hughes. She remembers her mother as being a strong disciplinarian. As she relayed this memory, Claire's voice was tinged with respect and perhaps longing for a time from the past when they were together. Those times were not necessarily special events but just part of everyday family living. For example, during meals, "once pule was done and the poi calabash [bowl] was uncovered, she learned from her mother and adopted grandmother that it was important to use the fingers to take only what you needed and to keep the calabash clean, without any track marks of residual poi around the edges." When the poi bowl was uncovered, her mother commanded Claire and her siblings to "not play, not fight, not cry" in order to show appreciation and respect for the foods, especially poi, and regard for the ways of our ancestors. It appears that Claire learned more from her mother than cultural protocol and ways, as she acknowledges that she too has a reputation for being strong-willed and a disciplinarian, especially in her role as an advocate for Hawaiian health.

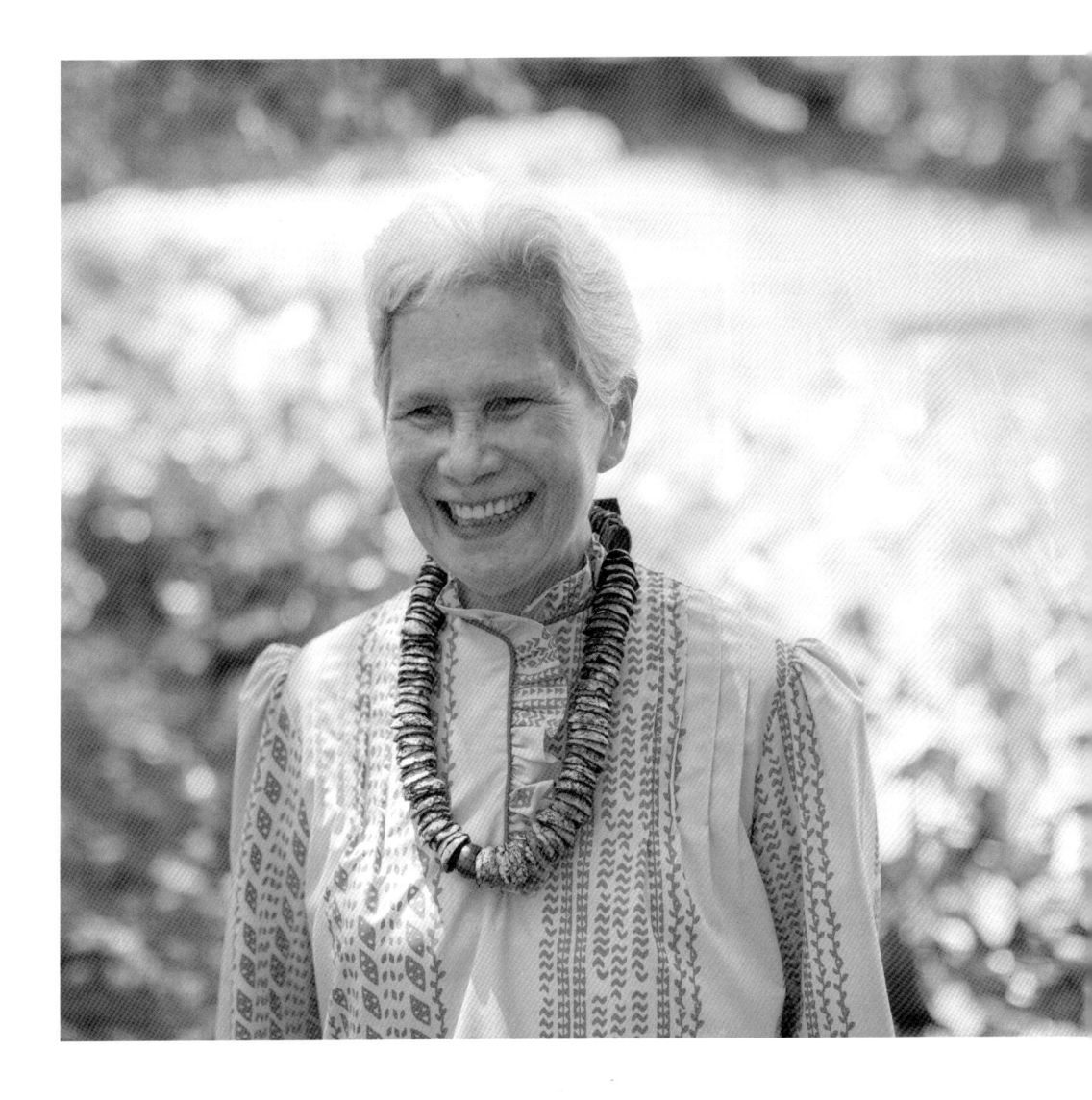

As she works and teaches people today about eating healthy, Claire shares the lessons from her elders. These family lessons are enriched by her higher education and knowledge of 'ai kapu and the protocol of food during ancient times, her collaborative work with colleagues equally committed to health and 'aiaola, and her experiences with people. Her learning and teaching are lifelong, and it is explicitly clear that Claire has a profound respect for the ways of our ancestors and recognizes that while some food traditions cannot work today, others may prove to be our best solutions.

Her life's work has earned her numerous prestigious awards that specifically recognize her achievements in nutrition and broadly acknowledge her accomplishments in Hawaiian culture. With humility, she credits family and colleagues for the awards. These tributes include the Living Treasures of Hawaiʻi Award from Honpa Hongwanji Mission in 2011, the ʻŌʻō Award from the Native Hawaiian Chamber of Commerce in 2012, the Nā Wāhine Puʻuwai Aloha Award from the Hawaiian Civic Club of Honolulu in 2016, and the David Malo Award from the Rotary Club of West Honolulu in 2017.

Claire also is well known for her health column in *Ka Wai Ola,* the newspaper of the Office of Hawaiian Affairs. In a 2019 column she wrote, "The remedies to return to the vibrant state of health of our ancestors are simple, although not necessarily easy. Making some small dietary changes and gradually adding physical activity will be rewarding and life-sustaining" (Hughes 2019, 12).

With her background in nutrition and public health, Claire is quick to acknowledge the important role of health advocates trained in different disciplines. Nutritionists, public health workers, physicians, social workers with a background in health, and community health workers are well equipped to address disease and disability. But Claire suggests that the related issues in the social, spiritual, and psychological domains of human functioning might also be addressed by social workers. For example, if the behaviors of excessive eating and drinking are linked to "filling the emptiness within," then perhaps counseling is warranted. Or if lack of a healthy diet is linked to lack of access to food choices, then perhaps improved social and economic advocacy and policies improving the availability and affordability of healthy foods in high-density Hawaiian communities are required.

Claire invites all those committed to Hawaiian health to work together. She continues to assert that building upon a traditional Hawaiian diet, or modification thereof, may help us reduce obesity and obesity-related disease. The traditional Hawaiian diet is primarily plant-based, with nutrients from foods such as taro, sweet potato, and limu kala, as well as protein from fish and some chicken and fowl. She cautions that knowing about healthy eating is not enough; to implement change we must apply what we know.

In looking to the past, Claire says that "if our ancestors didn't take care of their bodies, they couldn't plant, harvest, or prepare the taro for consumption," and they couldn't take care of themselves, their families, or aliʻi. In looking at the present and future, she says that if we don't take care of our bodies, we cannot take care of our own health and the welfare of our families and communities. Her philosophy for change is anchored in her principles and her belief in ancestral ways, combined with the reality of today's ever-changing society. Our way forward is, in part, to look back at history, appreciate the ways of our ancestors, and knowingly and respectfully apply those traditions to our lives today.

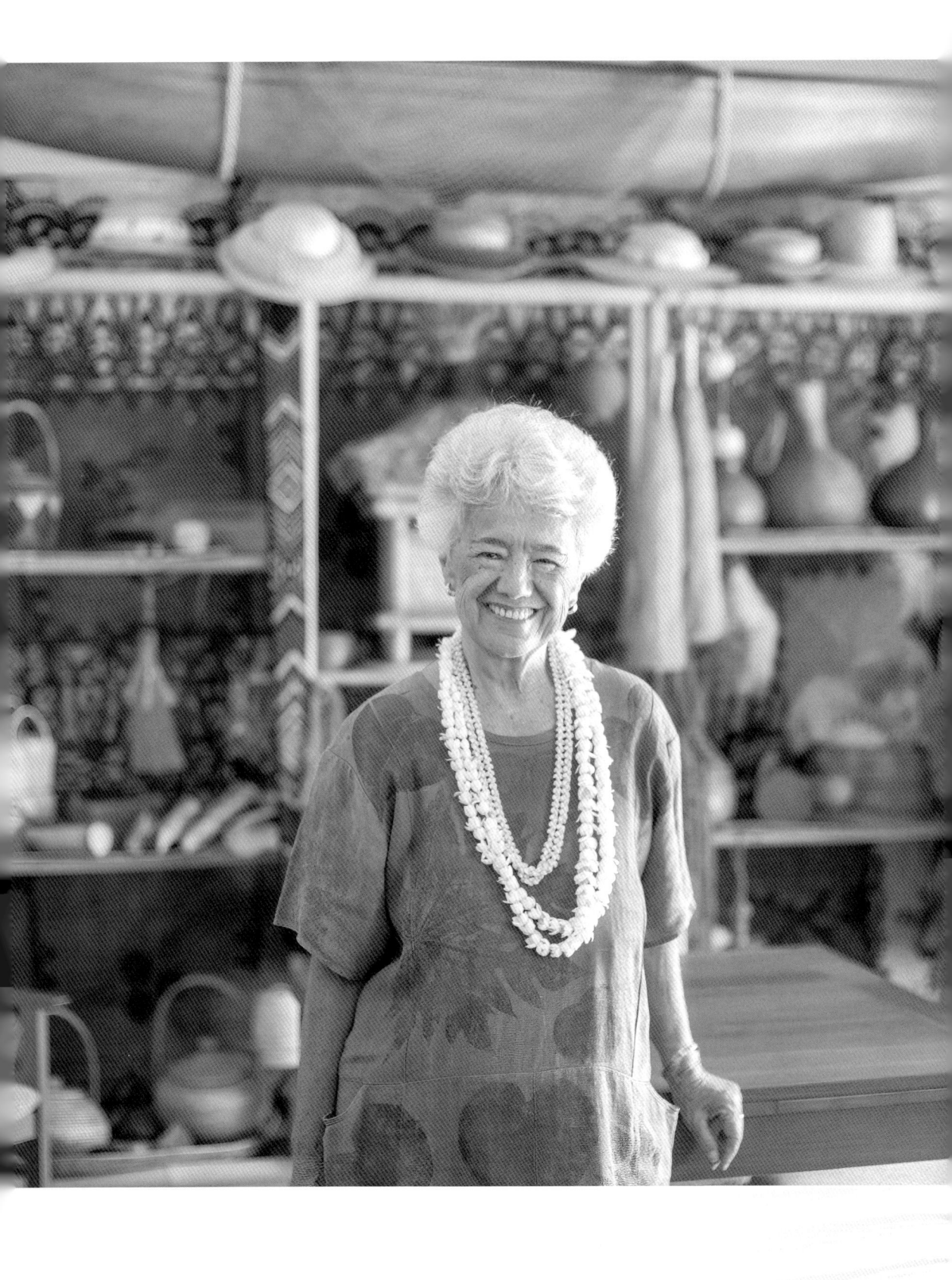

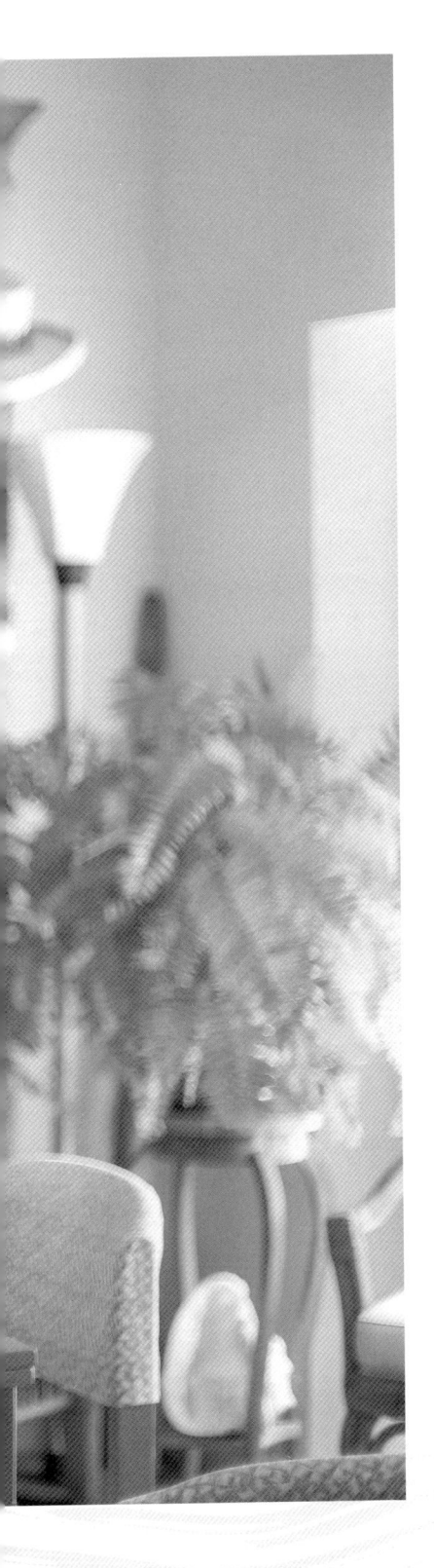

CHAPTER 6

Sarah Patricia ʻIlialoha Ayat Keahi

ʻŌLELO HAWAIʻI

Sarah Patricia ʻIlialoha Ayat Keahi, known to most as Kumu Keahi or Kumu Quick, held the kuleana of kumu ʻōlelo Hawaiʻi (Hawaiian language teacher) at Kamehameha Schools' (KS) Kapālama campus from 1966 to 2003. In nearly forty years of teaching, Sarah inspired thousands of young Native Hawaiian students in her creative teaching style of ʻōlelo Hawaiʻi. Many kumu ʻōlelo Hawaiʻi we know today, who are at the helm of the Hawaiian language movement, were once haumāna of Sarah and continue to speak words of endearment and aloha for her influence during their early years.

Sarah exudes an honest warmth that is undeniably palpable. Her presence transports you back in time to when the practice of hoʻokipa (hospitality) and haʻi moʻolelo (storytelling) were pillars of Hawaiian society. She takes the time to draw connections, to engage in shared stories, to share a few stories of her own, to put you at ease, and to welcome you into her space.

The title of kumu ʻōlelo Hawaiʻi was not one that Sarah would have associated herself with for most of her young life. Becoming one of the most well-known, loved, and respected Hawaiian language teachers was not something she aspired to be, because, in all honesty, the teaching of ʻōlelo Hawaiʻi was nonexistent in public or private schools in her youth.

Imprint of Family Influence

Sarah grew up during the 1950s and 1960s, and was reared for most of her childhood on the slopes of Papakōlea, one of the Hawaiian Homelands areas on the island of Oʻahu. Sarah is one of ten siblings, with four sisters and five brothers. Her interest in the Hawaiian language and love of mea Hawaiʻi (Hawaiian things) began early in her childhood and seemed to set her apart from her siblings. As she reminisces, Sarah fondly recalls a childhood memory of her relationship with her maternal grandmother, Sarah Keahi Kaʻōʻō Smythe, saying, "As a little girl, I was the one that sat at her knees and listened to her stories." Sarah states that her grandmother, who was originally from ʻUalapuʻe Molokaʻi but moved to Oʻahu and eventually settled with her family in Papakōlea, "lived from the time of the monarchy when Kalākaua was King, through the provisional government, the Republic, Territory, and ten years into statehood." Sarah recounts fond memories of everyday life with her grandmother, and with her mother, Helen Kauluwehiokalani Smythe Ayat, as they participated in featherwork, food preparation, hula, chanting, singing, and walaʻau (talking) with friends. Sarah loved listening to her kūpuna talk with her friends in Hawaiian. Each word effortlessly rolled off their tongues. They would string together a lei of sounds that, to Sarah, sounded like the beautiful melodies of the forest birds.

HE MEHEUHEU MAI NA KŪPUNA.

Habits acquired from ancestors.

(PUKUI 1983, 89)

These activities would shape Sarah's identity as a Native Hawaiian woman, educator, and advocate for the Hawaiian language.

Euphonious and Poetic Language

The Hawaiian language, like most Polynesian languages, is an oral one, rich in moʻolelo, kaʻao (legends), oli, and various kinds of mele. Sarah shared three aho (cords) through which the perpetuation of cultural practices, principles, and protocol were entwined directly into Hawaiian life: (a) moʻolelo and kaʻao; (b) mele and oli; and (c) ʻōlelo noʻeau and ʻōlelo nane (riddles, parables, allegories). She notes that societies of oral traditions primarily rely on memory, recall, and transference as a means to preserve their cultural heritage. The elders of oral communities such as those in Hawaiʻi become living sources of ʻōlelo, moʻomeheu (culture), and mōʻaukala (history) with the kuleana of transference to the younger generations.

The first aho includes moʻolelo and kaʻao. Both provide a foundational understanding from which Native Hawaiians can explore and express who they are (Goodyear-Kaʻōpua 2015). Stories and legends highlight the interconnectedness of all things and illuminate the ancestral knowledge that affirms Native Hawaiian identity both as individuals and as a community (Benham 2007). Figurative language is often skillfully woven into stories and legends through metaphors that conceal and reveal multiple layers of meaning. The layering of meanings, thoughts, and ideas is central to the Hawaiian language and plays an important role in the way that Native Hawaiians interpret and understand the world around them. Sarah says, "Just because you know the story or legend as it is presented literally does not necessarily mean that you know the metaphorical, and often hidden[,] meanings." Context, intent, and even physical location can give subtle hints as to other possible interpretations. The listener's established relationship with the speaker and his or her knowledge of a topic largely determines the degree to which the figurative language is understood (Oliveira 2019). Stories and legends hold within them many lessons on balance, relationships, and how to mālama all things living and not living, seen and unseen.

The second aho includes mele and oli. According to Pukui and Elbert (1986), a "mele" means a song or chant of any kind, a poem, poetry, to sing, or chant. Ordinary and extraordinary events, people, places, and things were recorded in mele. On the surface, the words of a mele can sometimes sound like something out of a modern-day superhero fable. Upon closer examination, the interpretation of the words reveal the hidden lessons embedded within each line. Sarah notes that "mele had various levels of meaning that may be shrouded by the ostensible literal meaning." An example of a mele in which the literal meaning is obvious would be one that "has a topographical meaning, like a song about a wahi pana and its surroundings." Others have a "historical or mythological meaning" that is metaphorical and speaks to different values of Hawaiian society, such as balance, reverence, and honor.

Whether literal or figurative, the lessons derived from mele were for Hawaiians indicators on how to live in harmony within their environment.

The third aho consists of ʻōlelo noʻeau and ʻōlelo nane. According to Sarah, these include "wise sayings and riddles," which may contain layers of meaning, from literal to figurative. When Sarah was growing up, ʻōlelo noʻeau were tools used in everyday life that provided opportunities for the transfer of knowledge from teacher to student and from kupuna to keiki (child). Sarah notes, "ʻŌlelo noʻeau give us insight into the thinking of our people . . . their worldview and what was important to them." Take the following ʻōlelo noʻeau about learning, for example:

Nānā ka maka; hoʻolohe ka pepeiao; paʻa ka waha.

Observe with the eyes; listen with the ears; shut the mouth.

(Pukui 1983, 248)

This proverb encourages one to observe and pay attention to one's whole being, while also promoting patience. It speaks to expectations and a way of knowing how to be.

Another example that informs us about learning is:

Ma ka hana ka ʻike.

In working one learns.

(Pukui 1983, 227)

This proverb is a beautiful successor to the former, meaning that once a period of observation and inquiry have passed, one can begin "doing." There is an emphasis on observation, as well as on learning through doing. In many ways, it contrasts with modern Western styles of learning through reading and writing.

Working through ʻōlelo nane is one of Sarah's favorite exercises with her students. ʻŌlelo nane are linguistic brain teasers that often hold hidden meanings. ʻŌlelo nane are used to show one's mental athleticism, quick wit, and proficiency in mea Hawaiʻi, and require both the speaker and interpreter to have a deep understanding of the language and of the Hawaiian worldview.

The following is one of Sarah's favorite 'ōlelo nane:

'EKOLU PĀ A LOA'A KA WAI.

Three walls, and you reach water.

(BECKWITH 1922, 312)

The answer is niu (coconut). The first pā (wall) is the husk, the second pā is the shell, and the third is the meat. Once you get through the three walls, you reach water. Sarah explains that one reason she enjoys sharing this 'ōlelo nane is because many people consider kumu niu (coconut trees) to be the most valuable plant in the Pacific.

All three aho are language-transmission practices. While rooted in antiquity, these 'ōlelo no'eau, mele, and 'ōlelo nane embody life lessons that transcend time and space, connecting Native Hawaiians directly to the source of their ancestral knowledge.

Pathway to Literacy

With the arrival of the first Christian missionaries in 1820 and King Liho-liho's (Kamehameha II) support of the value of literacy for his people, Native Hawaiians began learning to read and write in English (Laimana 2011). After just one year of instruction, a handful of pupils, all of whom were of the ali'i class, had developed such great skill that they were selected to teach English to fellow Hawaiians. By 1822, a pī'āpā (alphabet book) for 'ōlelo Hawai'i and elementary reading primers were created, printed, and distributed by the thousands. There was a rapid acquisition of reading and writing by young Hawaiian children. By 1825, close to 90 percent of the Hawaiian population had a pī'āpā book, and by 1834, close to 95 percent of Native Hawaiians were literate in 'ōlelo Hawai'i (Laimana 2011). Between 1834 and 1948, more than one hundred different Hawaiian-language nūpepa were published (Lorenzo-Elarco 2019).

Due to the efforts of Dwayne Nakila Steele and Dr. Puakea Nogelmeier, along with fluent scholarly interns, access to a large portion of the repository of nūpepa is accessible on the World Wide Web (Awaiaulu 2011). This repository continues to have great relevance for Hawaiians today. "Nūpepa shed light on not only the content but the content producers, demonstrating our long history of Hawaiian intellectualism. They also act as a conduit of ʻike that connects us to our past and allows us to communicate with our ancestors," says Sarah.

An Unexpected Calling

Sarah graduated from Roosevelt High School in 1962 and was accepted to the University of Hawaiʻi at Mānoa (UHM) to be trained as a teacher. The presence of Hawaiians on campus at that time was nominal at best. Her interest in the Hawaiian language prompted her to enroll in Hawaiian-language courses, which at the time were taught by Dr. Samuel H. Elbert, Pua Anthony, Sarah Nakoa, Kalani Meinecke, and later Dorothy Kahananui. One day after class, Dr. Elbert posed a question to Sarah that would change her life forever.

"What are you going to do after you graduate? Have you thought about it?" he asked.

Sarah said, "Well, I want to be a teacher!"

Dr. Elbert replied, "Oh, good, good, good. What kind of teacher?"

"Well, I'm thinking English," Sarah said enthusiastically.

"English?" he said surprisingly. "Do you know how many English teachers there are? Have you considered Hawaiian?"

"Hawaiian?" Sarah exclaimed, "I don't know ANY school that teaches Hawaiian!"

Dr. Elbert looked at Sarah with a bright gleam in his eye and replied, "There will be a day."

From that moment, Sarah knew and accepted her kuleana—to become a Hawaiian-language teacher. "I took everything in Hawaiian, all the classes, anything related to Hawaiian studies," she recounts. While an undergraduate, Sarah was privileged to be hired by the Bishop Museum to work in the recording lab with Eleanor Lilihana Aʻi Horswill Williamson. Elie, as most called her, accompanied Mary Kawena Pukui across the state, interviewing Native speakers, one of whom was Sarah's kupuna wahine (grandmother), Sarah Keahi Kaōʻō Smythe. Sarah's years at the Bishop Museum would prove to be invaluable in her future teaching career.

As Sarah began her final semester of student teaching, she received a telephone call from Dr. Donald Kilolani Mitchell, a teacher at Kamehameha Schools (KS) who was a strong supporter and advocate for Hawaiian culture. He was instrumental in starting Hui ʻŌiwi, a club for KS boys in 1931 that allowed students to study and practice Hawaiian cultural traditions (Eyre

2004). Dr. Mitchell was later appointed as the head of the Hawaiian Culture Committee at KS, which recommended that aspects of Hawaiian culture be incorporated into the curriculum. Sarah recalls her phone conversation with Dr. Mitchell.

"Hello! Is this Sarah Ayat?" Dr. Mitchell asked.

"Yes," Sarah answered with hesitancy.

"You don't know who I am, but I know who you are," said the voice on the other end. "My name is Don Mitchell, and I understand that you're ready to do student teaching in the Hawaiian language. I would like you to come to Kamehameha Schools."

"Well," Sarah exclaimed, "I'm scheduled to go to Farrington."

"Oh, I know," Dr. Mitchell said. "I already talked to your advisor, and she said if it's okay with you, you could come to KS."

As unexpected as the call seemed, it set Sarah on the path of teaching 'ōlelo Hawai'i and sharing the mo'olelo, mele, and everything learned from her kūpuna wahine, kumu, and many others along her road. She completed her student teaching at KS in May 1966, graduated from UHM in June, and was hired as a full-time teacher of the Hawaiian language in September.

Since the establishment of KS in 1887, the attitude toward the teaching of 'ōlelo Hawai'i underwent several changes. The use of the Hawaiian language was banned by its first principal, William Oleson. The school initially saw itself as an English immersion school, and immersion is the most powerful of language pedagogies (Eyre 2004). Oleson's successor, Theodore Richards, had a great appreciation for Hawaiian music and allowed Hawaiian songs to be included in the glee club program. By 1900, students were encouraged to participate in noncurricular and extracurricular activities that taught culture, and throughout the early 1900s, many visiting speakers, most of whom were non-Hawaiian, encouraged students to practice their language and culture. However, even with the establishment of the KS Song Contest in the early 1920s, very few students singing in 'ōlelo Hawai'i understood what they were singing. In 1924, Lydia K. Aholo became the first formal instructor of Hawaiian language at KS, although she was supported for only one year (Eyre 2004). Before long, due to low enrollment, the courses were withdrawn.

Under John Wise, the Hawaiian language was once again offered as an elective in 1927. While this was a win for the Hawaiian language, there were still those within the school's administration who opposed the perpetuation of Hawaiian culture. By 1931, the newly appointed principal of the School for Boys had a new plan for education that did not include the

Hawaiian language as part of the curriculum. When the staff at the Bernice Pauahi Bishop Museum heard this announcement, they immediately arranged for students to take Hawaiian culture classes at the museum on a weekly basis. In the years that followed, Hawaiian language classes started, stopped, and started again. In 1944, conversational Hawaiian was introduced to the elementary and intermediate school children at KS, taught by Mary Kawena Pukui.

In 1957, the Pukui and Elbert *Hawaiian Dictionary* appeared. Then, in 1961, Hawaiian was added to the list of foreign languages available to students in the two upper schools. In 1965, a 175-page textbook, *E Pāpā-ʻōlelo Kākou,* was written by Mrs. Dorothy M. Kahananui and used in teaching Hawaiian language to ninth-grade students in the first of a three-year sequence.

In 1966, when Sarah began working at KS, she continued using Kahananui's text for levels one and two. The limited resource materials available for teaching the upper-level Hawaiian language classes led Sarah back to the Bishop Museum, where she had worked with the Hawaiian nūpepa archives. The Hawaiian language newspapers were the perfect resource material for her upper-level students. She was so excited to work alongside her students to translate these raw materials. "It was great and fascinating for me," she said, "because I was learning along with them. It was gratifying exposing and introducing our students to primary sources."

In 1973, almost half a century after Lydia K. Aholo was a short-term Hawaiian language instructor, Sarah and Dr. Mitchell's proposal was accepted to require high school students to take a semester each of Hawaiian history and culture. Sarah stated, "We proposed the requirement for six or seven years in a row . . . it was never accepted." Although this was a massive win at the time, it took many more years for the Hawaiian language proficiency requirement to follow suit. In 2014, KS announced that all students, beginning with the class of 2017, must demonstrate a level of Hawaiian language proficiency equivalent to that which could be acquired in a Hawaiian I Language course in high school. Students now must pass a Hawaiian language proficiency test that assesses four skill areas: listening, speaking, reading, and writing.

Cultivating the Future of the Hawaiian Language

"The inability to speak Hawaiian is considered a major personal cultural loss by many contemporary Hawaiians" (Wilson and Kamanā 2006, 157). Because nuances of Hawaiian ways of knowing and thinking are intricately woven into the grammar and vocabulary of the Hawaiian language, it has been challenging for contemporary Hawaiians to fully grasp the cultural and spiritual essence that reigned supreme in Hawaiʻi for thousands of years. The abundance of unique ancestral knowledge and creativity found in traditional forms of oratory and poetry remained out of reach. The strategic attempt to erase the Hawaiian language included various types of propaganda, whose intent was to instill doubt and fear and to coerce Hawaiians into questioning the lifestyle they had known. The notion during the late 1800s was that Hawaiian was an aboriginal language that ultimately hindered the ability of students to express the higher-order thinking necessary for an educated population. However, in sharp contrast to the popular belief, a nūpepa titled *Kūʻokoʻa* printed an editorial denouncing the claim of the inferiority of the Hawaiian language. The author cited the numerous Hawaiian-speaking judges, lawyers, teachers, publishers, and ministers practicing at that time, and predicted that the implementation of an English-medium education would lead to a reduction of academic achievement among Hawaiians (Wilson and Kamanā 2006).

Through the generations, the vibration of ancestral voices never ceased. They are beckoning Hawaiians to return to the source of knowledge, wisdom, and aloha that is ʻōlelo Hawaiʻi. The 1970s was a time of revival. The resurgence of Hawaiian culture and language gained momentum in Hawaiian communities. The cultural pride and the ferocious hunger for cultural knowledge paved the way for many positive changes that would come. By 1978, the president of the constitutional convention, John Waiheʻe, proposed that the Hawaiian language be accorded the status of official language, along with English, and that the study of Hawaiian be accorded special promotion by the state (Proceedings of the Constitutional Convention of Hawaii of 1978 1980). Both provisions passed, catapulting the Hawaiian Renaissance movement forward and breathing life into a Hawaiian-language immersion program in preschool through ʻAha Pūnana Leo (ʻAPL) in 1984. Concerned ʻAPL parents urged the Hawaiʻi Department of Education (HIDOE) to extend Hawaiian-language education to the public school system for their children matriculating from the ʻAPL preschools. The department heard the call and began its efforts to build a continuum of Hawaiian-language immersion through a pilot program during the 1987–1988 school year with funding provided by the Native Hawaiian Education Act. Since then, the Hawaiian Language Immersion Program, as it was named, has continued to grow, currently overseeing twenty-two HIDOE sites and six charter school sites on six of the eight populated islands (Hawaiʻi State Department of Education n.d.).

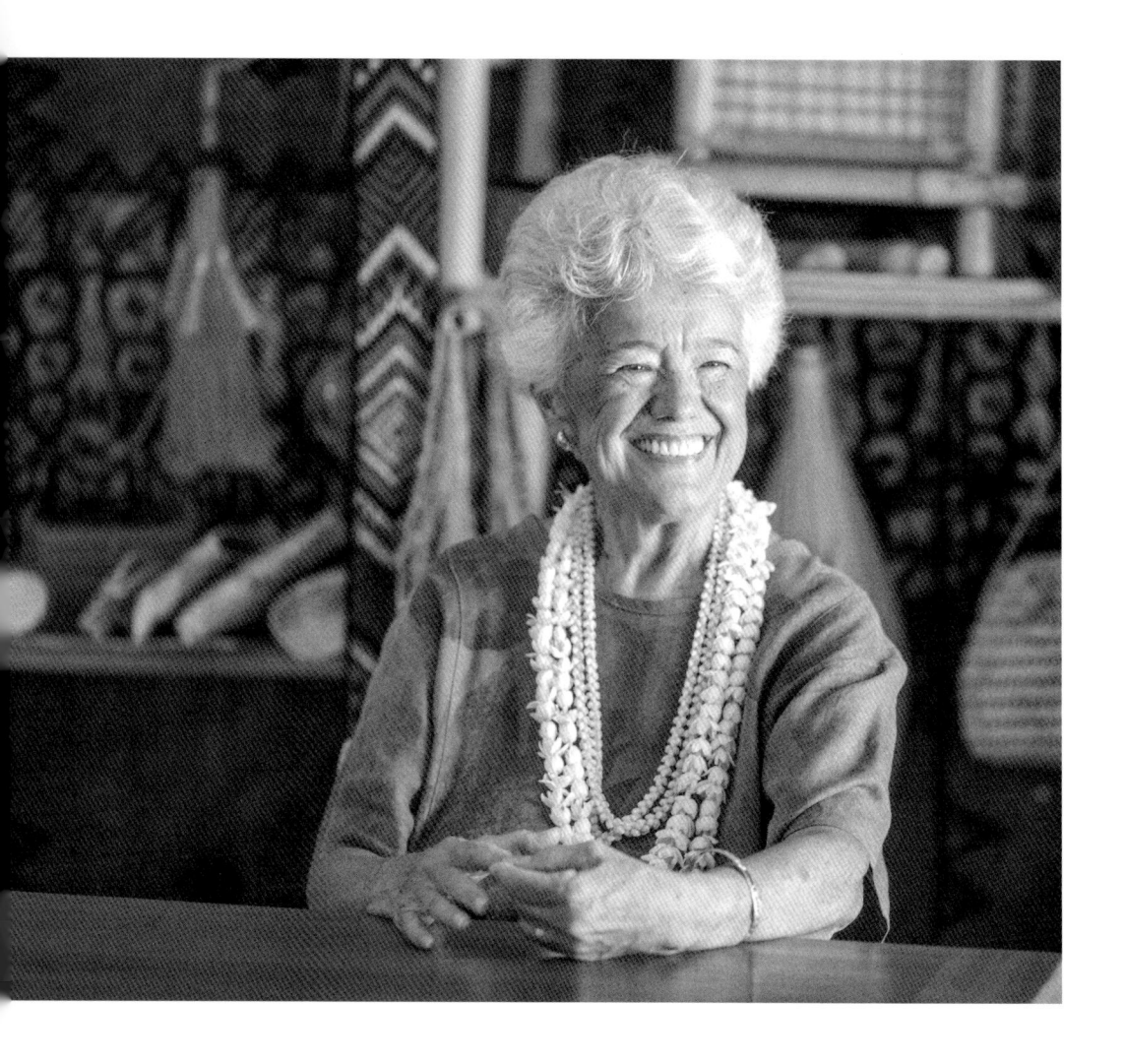

When asked about the future of ʻōlelo Hawaiʻi, Sarah's response was optimistic: "Hawaiians today have many more ways to access this and other types of ancestral knowledge, primarily through the use of technology. For example, we have Duolingo. We have the OHA newspaper, *Ka Wai Ola,* which includes a section of haʻawina ʻōlelo Hawaiʻi (Hawaiian language lessons). This section teaches lessons on sentence structure, vocabulary words, and easy conversational patterns. Hawaiʻi Public Radio has its Hawaiian word of the day."

In addition, there are more and more opportunities for families and individuals to participate in everyday events and activities hosted by

Hawaiian-language organizations and speakers. For example, in 2018, a collaboration between Ke Keʻena Hoʻonaʻauao Hawaiʻi, Kanaeokana, the Department of Education, and EK Fernandez hosted Pō ʻŌlelo Hawaiʻi, Hawaiian language night at the kāniwala, or carnival. The event was intended to create and encourage ʻōlelo spaces where the Hawaiian language can be perpetuated through interactions among speakers of all levels. Over five thousand people attended the event and got a chance to experience what it would be like for the Hawaiian language to be the everyday language (Kanaeokana n.d.).

Sarah teaches us that "language is the vehicle by which culture and history are transmitted. With fundamental awareness and understanding of language, we bring forth ancestral knowledge that provides a foundation from which social justice and health equity can be actualized." She shares one of her favorite sayings that captures her personal journey as a language teacher. This saying renders a clear message to all Hawaiians, encouraging them to learn, preserve, and perpetuate the ways of their ancestors, to be proud of who they are and where they come from, and to honor and acknowledge the wisdom that came through thousands of years of observations and trials. She states,

> E HELE WĀWAE KĀKOU E LIKE ME KO KĀKOU,
> KŪPUNA ME KE KAPUKAPU A ME KA HAʻAHEO.
>
> *Let us walk like our ancestors, with dignity and pride.*

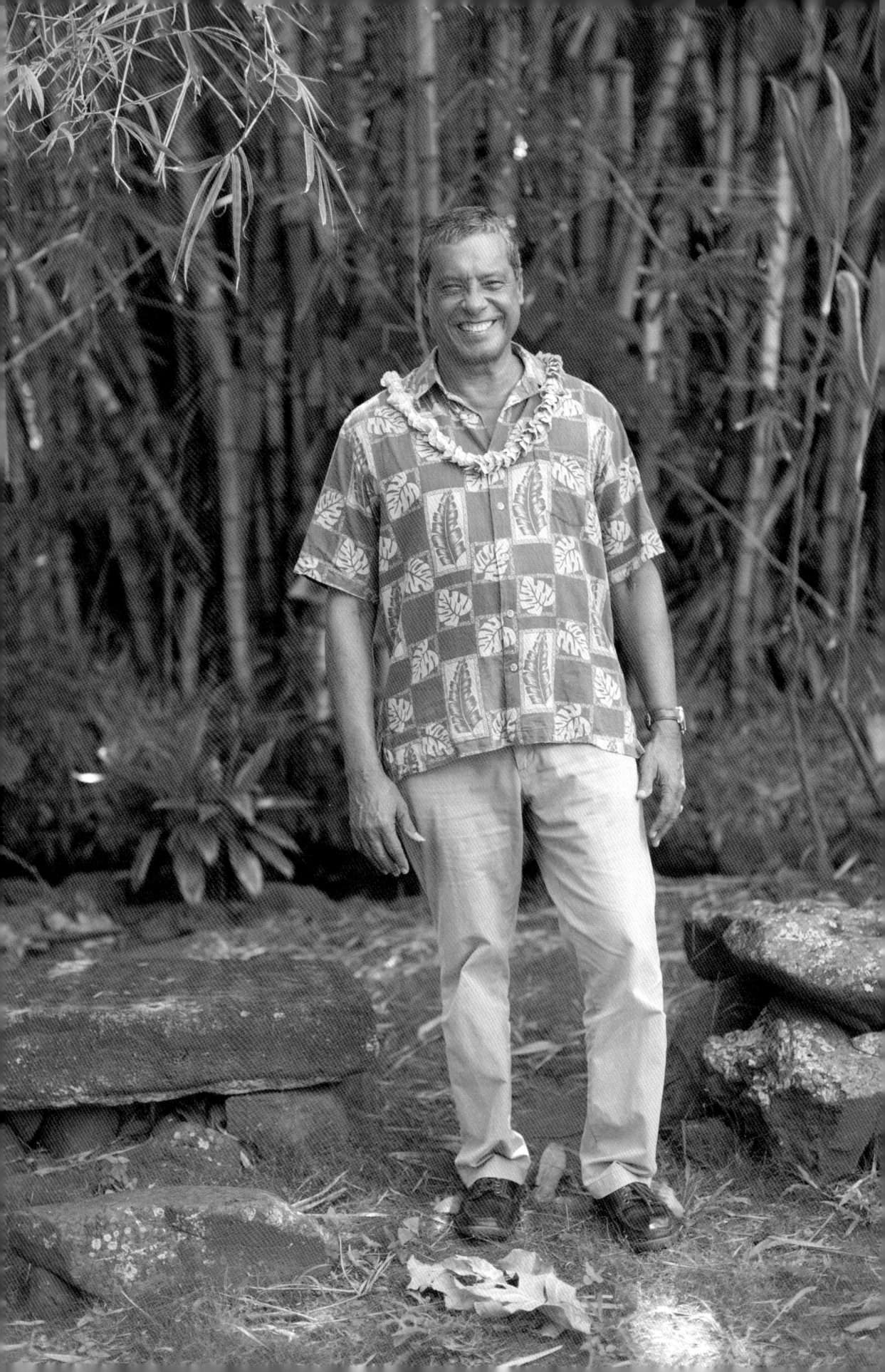

CHAPTER 7

Jonathan Kay Kamakawiwoʻole Osorio

MELE

Jonathan Kay Kamakawiwoʻole Osorio is an activist who has artfully blended his advocacy for Hawaiian self-determination with mele that address humanity and the restoration of justice. He teaches others about the role of mele in documenting events, conveying important messages, bringing people together, and making us human. He also is an academic scholar and leader at the University of Hawaiʻi at Mānoa (UHM), serving as professor and dean of the Hawaiʻinuiākea School of Hawaiian Knowledge. His life's work is heavily reliant on the power of words, and in many of his talks, he is quick to note the importance of words, as illustrated in the following ʻōlelo noʻeau:

> ### I KA ʻŌLELO NO KE OLA, I KA ʻŌLELO NO KA MAKE.
>
> *Life is in speech; death is in speech.*
>
> (Pukui 1983, 129)

Based on his mastery in mele, Osorio was awarded a Lifetime Achievement Award from the Hawaiʻi Academy of Recording Arts in 2019. In accepting the award, he acknowledged that music will always be a part of his life and "that for Kānaka Maoli, composing, performing, singing, and hula are things that have kept us alive as a people through some very difficult times" ("Lifetime Achievement Award" 2019). Says Jon,

Mele means music, and for Kānaka Maoli, all mele have lyrics. Although we have famous instrumentalists in our lāhui, in general, that's not what we do when we create music, when we haku [braid] mele, which means to compose songs. We sing lyrics, which are poetry. And the melody, rhythm, and lyrics are entwined like a haku [braided] lei to create a song. Mele appeals to more than the intellect. It appeals to that emotive spiritual sense of self. It is more than someone giving a speech, although a mele can contain important content. It also connects people and sends a message that lodges in your naʻau [mind, heart, gut].

Music as Destiny

Jon was born on the island of Hawaiʻi. His paternal great-grandfather was Charles Moses Kamakawiwoʻole from Kamuela, and his paternal great-grandmother was Daisy Kaaiawaawa from Kukaiau, a very narrow ahupuaʻa in Hāmākua. His great-grandfather was descended from a line of chiefs who were hana lawelawe (serving chiefs) to King Kamehameha. The strength of the relationship of service to Kamehameha is reflected in the family name of Kamakawiwoʻole o Kamehameha, which means "of or with Kamehameha," rather than Kamakawiwoʻole a Kamehameha, which means "belonging to."

The significance of names in Hawaiian culture is profound. Jon's paternal grandmother, Eliza Kamakawiwoʻole, named him and all of his siblings, Jon's firstborn, the two children born to his older brother, and the four children born to his older sister. Jon and his son Kanealiʻi were chosen to carry the family name of Kamakawiwoʻole. In Hawaiian culture, bestowing an inoa kupuna (ancestral name) is a form of honoring and perpetuating lineage and legacy, as captured in this ʻōlelo noʻeau:

OLA KA INOA.

The name lives.

(PUKUI 1983, 272)

Although he is not sure why the name was not passed on to his older siblings, Jon acknowledges the significance of Hawaiian names in according kuleana. The name Kamakawiwoʻole connotes "fearlessness," and one might interpret this as appropriate for a person whose trajectory in life reflects a deep commitment to activism and social justice.

Jon's first experiences with music were at home and in church. At a very young age, Jon showed musical talent by singing different harmonies when other people were singing melody during Sunday church services. At the age of seven, Jon's father, an accomplished guitar player, enrolled Jon in 'ukulele lessons with Harriet "Danby" Walker Beamer, a well-known kumu hula, dancer, composer, and singer in Hilo. On cool, misty Saturday mornings in Hilo, Jon learned to play the 'ukulele in a small class of other seven- and eight-year olds, including Keola and Kapono Beamer. He mastered a number of Hawaiian songs. But he was surrounded by Western music, and he quickly looked for ways to use the 'ukulele to accompany Western songs.

Jon boarded at Kamehameha Schools in Honolulu from the age of twelve, and there he met other young Hawaiians playing rock and roll and American folk music on the 'ukulele and the guitar, including his dormitory mate, Jerry Santos, who later founded the singing group Olomana: "Even though we were getting this amazing education in mele, singing mele in Glee Club, and singing mele at song contests, we were interested in using 'ukulele and guitar with Western and American folk music." Jon picked up the guitar in his junior year and started to write his own songs to express himself in English.

Although many of Jon's Kamehameha classmates were interested in Hawaiian music, Jon admits that, at first, he was not that attracted to playing it. But then he heard The Sunday Mānoa, a musical group started in the 1960s by Peter Moon, Palani Vaughan, Cyril Pahinui, and Albert "Baby" Kalima Jr. In 1971, the group was reconstituted with Peter Moon and Roland and Robert Cazimero, and their 1971 album *Guava Jam* was later hailed as a marker of the start of the Hawaiian Renaissance (Berger 1994). Jon recalls, "You could hear what you could do with a guitar and with rhythm . . . that you could take old songs and make them incredibly lively in the way that our music was lively at the time." He remembers being immediately sold. He started combining mele that were thirty, forty, fifty, and sixty years old with American folk music. This led him to composing music with themes related to Hawaiian identity and advocacy.

Mele as a Platform for Change

Mele can be a powerful avenue for the expression of social and political ideology. Jon says that many Hawaiian musical artists in the 1960s and 1970s were using Hawaiian music as a platform for making statements about the condition of Hawaiians in our homeland. He states, "It was not just about issues of poverty and undereducation but about deep emotional issues, like a people being lost." Jon believes that mele can help Native Hawaiians, who were subjected to intense assimilation following Western contact, to "reconnect again and begin to see themselves as really belonging together."

In the mid-1970s, Jon started writing and playing music with Randy Borden. Their group, known as Jon & Randy, became a major player in the Hawaiian music scene in the 1970s and was the opening act for concerts featuring musicians from the continental United States, including Leo Kottke, the Jacksons, and Tower of Power. In 1981, Jon and Randy won a Nā Hōkū Hanohano Award (the Hawaiian equivalent of a Grammy) for "Hawaiian Eyes," a song about a people that had lost themselves in American culture and were trying to find a way back.

HAWAIIAN EYES

Often in the darkness, sometimes in the light
Visions of your golden eyes, sparkle in my sight.
Haunted by those graceful years,
when we were young and life was sharp and clear.

Can you see me now, Hawaiian eyes?
Can you see me lost from paradise?
There were so many ways to go
So many things to know
But I've missed you inside
Hawaiian eyes.

Shouting in the mountains, silent by the stream
Our eyes held each other's, locked in secret dreams.
Now we're freed and drifting on,
memories of you hover still and strong.

In this period, Jon was heavily influenced by George Helm, a legendary activist of the aloha ʻāina movement. George also was a gifted musician who knew Hawaiian history and the language. Jon remembers George as being able to intricately weave stories about the circumstances of the Hawaiian people. Through his music, George would teach about the overthrow of the Hawaiian monarchy and about Kahoʻolawe, the island leeward of Maui and Molokaʻi that the US military used for bombing practice. Jon remembers, "My grandmother told me when I was really young that the navy bombed Kahoʻolawe, and she said the Hawaiian word ʻpohōʼ [damage] with great distain, implying the incredible waste of the island from this bombing." Because of George, Jon learned that the US military had been using the island of Kahoʻolawe for target practice since World War II and had detonated more than five hundred tons of explosives above and on the island, cracking the water table and allowing the island's freshwater supply to seep into the ocean (Osorio 2014).

George used his music to educate, appearing at churches, schools, and civic club meetings to talk about Kahoʻolawe and the need to take it back from the US military. Jon recalls a story about the power of song in education: "George went to Hilo to address the Hilo Hawaiian Civic Club, but he was not allowed on the agenda. So he stood outside the building where the meeting was taking place and started playing guitar and singing. And one by one everybody came out. And when they were all out, he began to talk about aloha ʻāina. So, through song, people can be drawn together, and anger and divisiveness set aside."

George Helm disappeared at sea during one of his attempts to occupy Kahoʻolawe as a way to protest the bombing. Jon and Randy wrote the song "Hawaiian Soul" in March 1977 on the day the search for George and another Kahoʻolawe activist, Kimo Mitchell, was called off. Neither was found. In recognizing George's role in a struggle to recapture the essence of being Native Hawaiian, this song touched a deep chord of loss and sparked activism among many Hawaiians.

HAWAIIAN SOUL

I can recall the way, your voice would fill the room
And we would all be stilled, by your melody
And now your voice is gone, and to the sea belongs
All of the gentle songs, that you had harbored

Hawaiian soul
How could you leave us
You've not been lost at sea
You're only wandering

Hawaiian soul
We sing your melody
And send them out to sea
You know the harmony

They say before you left, to seek your destiny
That older voices called, and drowned your laughter
But I believe you knew, what you would have to be
A beacon in the storm, to guide us after

Jon thinks the Hawaiian sovereignty movement, which started to develop at that time, is about restoring our faith in the law and its ability to restore justice and fairness. It is much less about acquiring resources and much more about protecting them and assuring the survival of these islands for the generations to come. He believes the movement was and continues to be about safeguarding the right of Native Hawaiians to live, speak, think, and behave as Hawaiians and to teach their children that they may be Hawaiian and not American. "I think that the Hawaiian sovereignty movement will ultimately produce a nation and government devoted to peace and disarmament, that carefully manages our lands and waters, and that protects the cultural diversity that has defined this place," he says.

Jon believes that mele and haku mele (to compose songs) have always played, and will continue to play, a strong role in the expression of truth, in the use and celebration of Hawaiian language, and in bringing people together toward a vision of full independence under a multiethnic nation-state that is culturally Hawaiian. In a tribute to the Hawaiian sovereignty movement, Jon and Randy, along with Steve Brown, set to music the "Pule No Ke Ea" (Prayer for Sovereignty) written by Kanalu Young to offer sovereignty as a solution to political oppression (Berger 1997; Young n.d.). The first verse:

E kāko'o mai
E ala,
Launa pū . . .
'O Mauna'ala
I ke Ea
Pā mai nei ka Lanakila ē
I mau mai ka mana'o

Show support
Wake up,
Gather as one . . .
Mauna'ala
In spirit
Wind blows
To further the feeling.

Value of History in Teaching Mele

In his thirties, Jon returned to school to study Hawaiian history, culture, and 'ōlelo Hawai'i. He recognized that to create mele as a statement for social justice, he needed to know more about Hawaiian history and to learn the Hawaiian language. He earned his PhD in history, became a faculty member of Hawaiian studies, and later became dean of the Hawai'inuiākea School of Hawaiian Knowledge at the UHM. He is proud that Hawai'inuiākea offers Hawaiian language courses and degrees and that kamali'i (children) have opportunities to learn 'ōlelo Hawai'i through Hawaiian-language immersion schools. Says Jon, "We didn't have these opportunities, and I didn't start to learn 'ōlelo Hawai'i until I was thirty-seven years old. Because of this, I do not understand the richness and all the symbols and references of this beautiful language."

Jon's teaching of advocacy through mele has benefited the many students who have taken classes from him. Jon draws on his background as a composer and singer, and his favorite course to teach is "Mele o Ke Hou: Music and Native Identity," which explores Hawaiian music as an avenue for social, cultural, and political expression—traditionally, historically, and in contemporary society. Traditionally, Hawaiians did not have a written language, so until the 1800s, mele and oli were the ways Hawaiians created and transmitted information about events, behaviors, feelings, and lessons: "The mele was the poetry of the chant. In the elaborate system of ancient days, life was a continuous ceremony, and there was an appropriate mele for every occasion" (Handy et al. 1965, 204).

Memorized mele and chants were long a reliable source of information about the past and present, and lessons from mele were used to inform decision making and to guide future action. Says Jon, "It is my belief that all of the mele—the genealogies of chiefs, homage to a particular rain or a particular place, a moʻolelo of lovers or enemies—were very intentionally composed to serve as journals and diaries." Jon is convinced that people who rely on oral (rather than written) language develop prodigious memories, as well as a deep appreciation for words and the use of words. He believes Western society has lost this because of its reliance on text.

In the early 1800s, Christian missionaries arrived and set the oral language of the islands down in text. King Liholiho (Kamehameha II) embraced the value of literacy, and in 1822 a pīʻāpā for ʻōlelo Hawaiʻi was written and broadly distributed. In 1834, it was estimated that close to 90 percent of Native Hawaiians were literate in ʻōlelo Hawaiʻi (Laimana 2011). Although reading and writing enabled Native Hawaiians to write down their views and histories, the late 1800s brought laws and policies that systematically dismantled the Native Hawaiian worldview. Music, however, was an element of the Hawaiian culture that withstood the waves of change.

As Jon noted in his 2019 course syllabus for "Hawaiian Studies 478: Mele o Ke Hou: Music and Native Identity," "The loss of the Hawaiian nation to American occupation in 1898 signaled a period of tremendous oppression of the Native culture and point of view in every way but for music. Even during the most politically repressive territorial years, Hawaiian composers continually represented a powerful and defiant Native persona that heralded the political and cultural explosiveness of the past 40 years" (Osorio 2019, 1).

Says Jon, "Mele documents the past, but it also helps Native Hawaiians today to reconnect to each other and to begin to see themselves as really belonging together." Jon teaches his students about mele as a form of communication that can signal defiance to oppression or commemorate a significant event. In class, he encourages students to work together to compose mele to convey information but also to build a community for expressing ideas through song. For example, students in his classes have written songs for Queen Liliʻuokalani and for activists for Mauna Kea. As he describes it, "Generally what happens is that somebody comes up with the melody, and then someone will take a line that we've crafted together, and we'll start to sing."

The Next Generation

Jon believes that we can return to a time when haku mele becomes as natural as breathing. "The impulse of 'writing as gift' is still very much with us as a

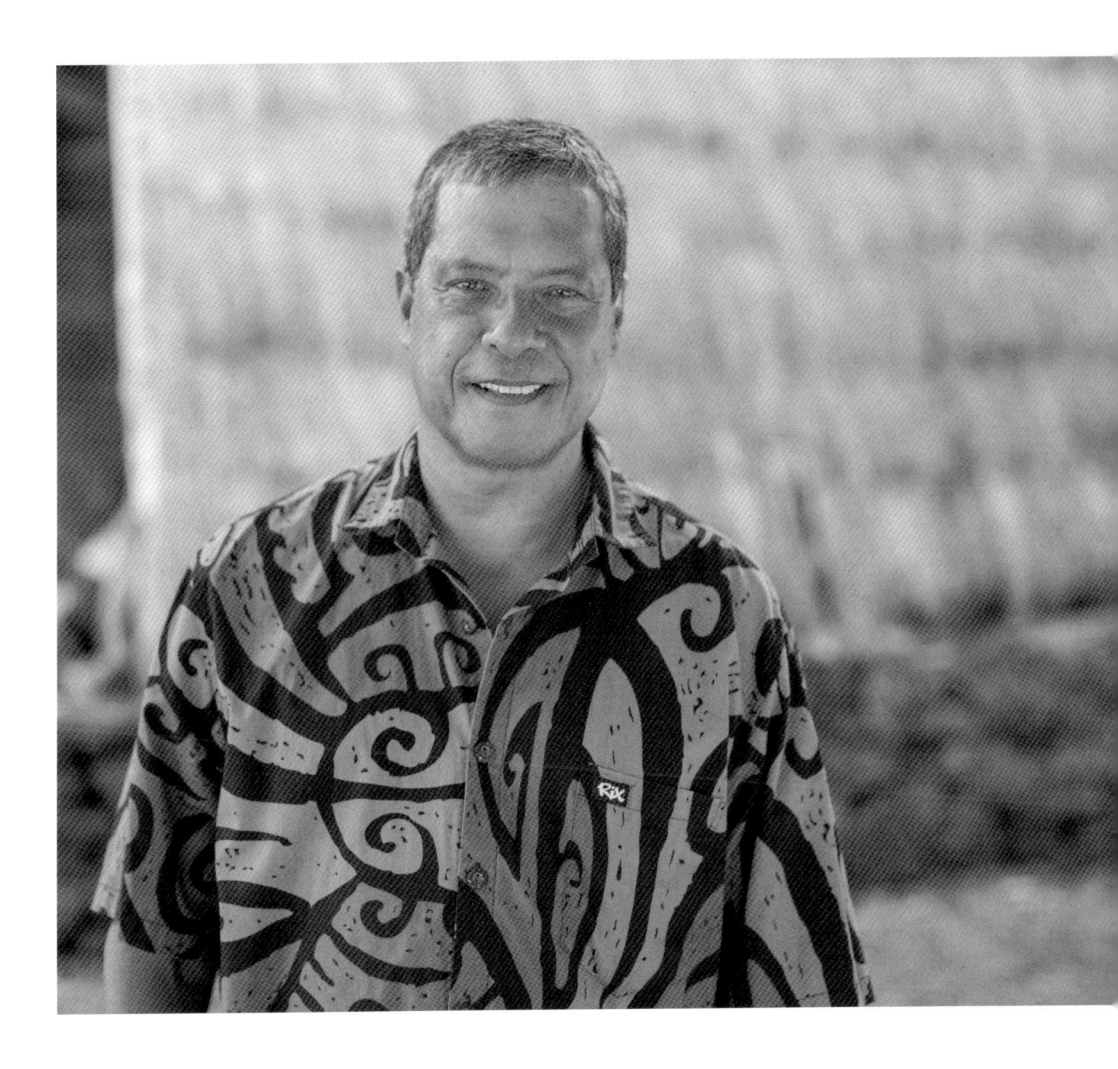

people today," he says. "So many of the songs that I wrote and I believe others in my generation wrote tried to express us as a people. I don't believe that they were done to give us a career or make us famous. I believe that they were done as gifts to our people sort of writ large." Jon himself has written mele as commemorative gifts. For example, he wrote a mele for his daughter Lehua when she was adopted, for his wife for one of her birthdays, and for Kamana Beamer's daughter when she celebrated her first birthday. He also composed "Hawaiian Spirits Live Again," a mele for his grandmother, Eliza Kamakawiwoʻole, that expresses deep ties to ʻāina and heritage. By gifting mele to one another, he says, "I think we're coming back to this notion of mele being something special we can do for other people and therefore give them something that is priceless."

Although Jon and many of his generation learned Hawaiian language and mele later in life, he sees members of the next generation who are very grounded in language and mele. For example, Kīhei de Silva has written numerous articles about mele and the references to places in Kailua, where he lives with his wife, Māpuana de Silva. In these articles, Kīhei writes with care about the kaona (hidden meaning) of each song, and this helps to enhance our understanding of the mele and the time in which it was written. The couple taught their children ʻōlelo Hawaiʻi and, one of them, Kahikina de Silva, is fluent in the Hawaiian language and its nuances. In this way, Hawaiʻi has a growing number of residents who were raised speaking Hawaiian and now have excellent command of the language. "This includes their ability to recognize the fullness of the word in its different contexts, how a word or phrase should be said, and the facial expressions to use when expressing a particular meaning of the word," Jon says.

Using ʻōlelo Hawaiʻi in mele is increasing with growing access to lessons and formal education in the Hawaiian language. At the university level, ʻōlelo Hawaiʻi and Hawaiian studies courses are among the most popular courses across the University of Hawaiʻi at Mānoa, the University of Hawaiʻi–West Oʻahu, the University of Hawaiʻi–Hilo, the University of Hawaiʻi Maui College, and University of Hawaiʻi community colleges. The establishment of Hawaiʻinuiākea as a school at the UHM will help assure that generations to come have the opportunity to acquire Hawaiian knowledge. In addition to courses in mele, courses are offered in Hawaiian language, history, law, sovereignty, protocol, chant, genealogy, literature, and ʻōlelo noʻeau, as well as in Hawaiian approaches to kalo cultivation and to land, ocean, and water management. Other courses teach about Indigenous research methods, lāʻau lapaʻau, Hawaiian fiber arts and printmaking, Hawaiian myth, hula, and other topics.

Jon also is excited to see a whole group of new Hawaiian composers writing in ʻōlelo Hawaiʻi. He identified only a handful of songwriters from the last century who composed what Jon calls "real mele." Now, says Jon, "when I hear the lyrics of the songwriters raised with Hawaiian language, I can hear their fluency. So, to me, there's no question that mele is going to continue." Also, students and faculty at Hawaiʻinuiākea are engaged in restoring the old mele, realizing that "forgetting or losing the mele from old Hawaiʻi would result in the loss of valuable cultural knowledge, poetic language usage, native expressions, place names, rain names, and so forth" (Lopes 2010).

Jon tells his students and other young people to continue to engage in music. "Whether it's haku mele, whether it's singing, whether it's performing, whether it's learning kīhōʻalu [Hawaiian slack key], or whether it's another creative endeavor, these are the things that give your life a vitality, regardless of what you are forced to do to make a living." He wishes governments understood the importance of public education in the creative arts and humanities. These subjects enhance our ability to express ourselves and to be able to document and transmit information about the beauty and evil around us and how it makes us feel. "The arts can inspire us as individuals and enhance our ability to inspire others. I'm convinced," Jon adds, "that this is what makes us human."

Jon feels that his musical career and his career as an educator are really the same thing: "When I got into music, it was because there were things Hawaiians wanted to communicate—the need to preserve what we had, look carefully to the future, and cherish those things left to us by our elders and ancestors." Jon feels that mele is a good vehicle for communicating these ideas, and he has dedicated his life to preserving and advancing mele as a Hawaiian cultural practice. He continues to educate young Hawaiians and others about mele and its important role in documenting events, bringing people together, making us human, and connecting us spiritually.

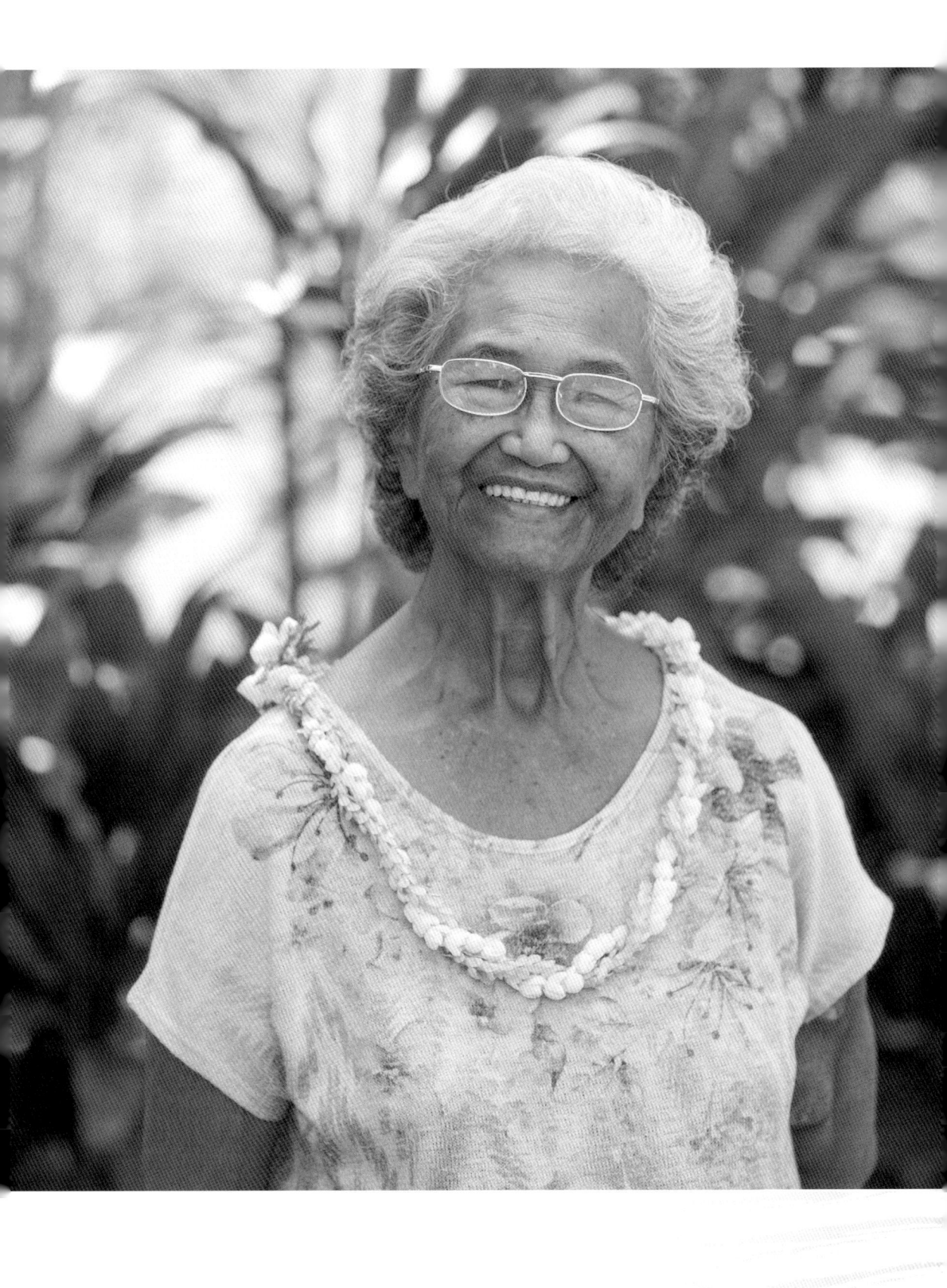

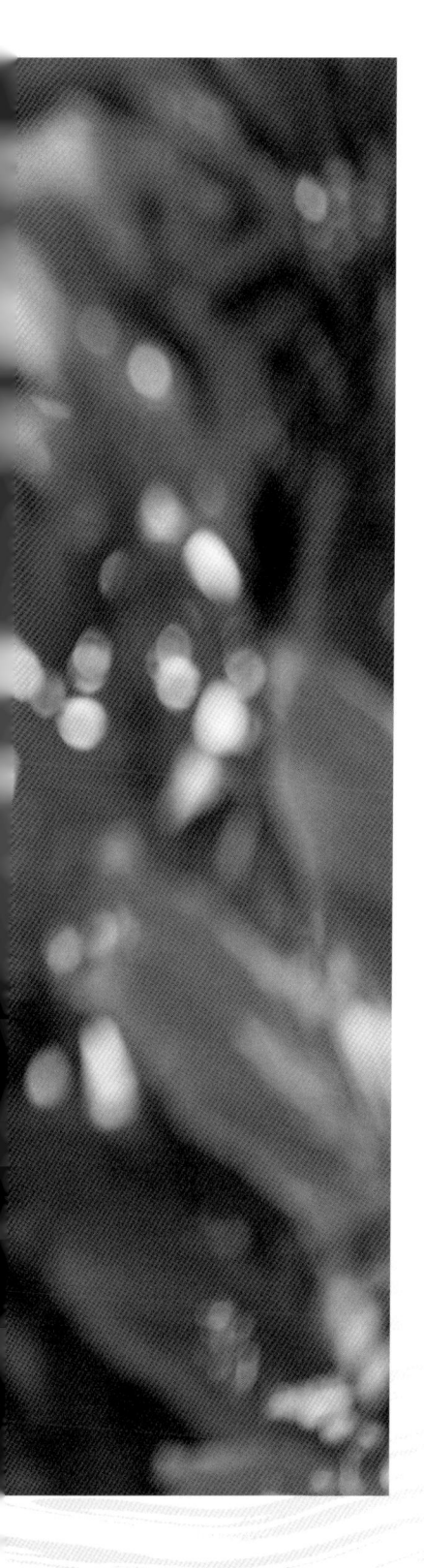

CHAPTER 8

Lynette Kaʻopuiki Paglinawan

HOʻOPONOPONO

Lynette Kaʻopuiki Paglinawan has dedicated a good portion of her life to cultivating and strengthening the well-being of Native Hawaiians and is renowned for her work in hoʻoponopono. Lynette's innate gift of engagement, steeped in the cultural wisdom and life experiences of her ʻohana, has provided a safe space for others to grow and transform. Her personal and professional commitment to others occurred through education, mentorship, and moʻolelo.

The Essence of Hawaiian Knowing and Being

Known affectionately to most as ʻAnakē (auntie), Lynette was born and raised in Pauoa and Nuʻuanu, Oʻahu. She grew up in the 1950s and 1960s and lived with her grandparents, who taught her cultural principles, practices, and protocol. Her grandparents emphasized that family practices and the essence of Hawaiian knowing and being were foundational to life. Lynette knows that her lifestyle sharply contrasts with many other Hawaiian families who experienced cultural losses as they adjusted to Western ways.

Many Hawaiian families lost touch with Hawaiian practices, took the practices into secrecy, or abandoned them altogether for fear of judgment, ridicule, and persecution (Pukui, Haertig, and Lee 1972). Lynette believes that cultural losses contributed to many of the social issues experienced by families today.

Her life's work is dedicated to strengthening the ʻohana by restoring cultural values such as love and loyalty to ʻohana, reverence for kūpuna, and respect for cultural traditions. The ʻohana is a group of people, joined by blood, marriage, and adoption, that shares a sense of unity, involvement, and responsibility (Pukui, Haertig, and Lee 1972). Members are interdependent and provide each other with assistance, emotional support, and resources. The concept of ʻohana implies solidity, cohesiveness, love, and loyalty among members. This is not to say that ʻohana members do not disagree or argue. To disagree is human, but disagreements should not break the ʻohana. Lynette states, "The maintenance of familial relationships is very important to the survival (physical, emotional, and spiritual) of the closely-knit unit and Hawaiian culture."

To strengthen Hawaiian families, Lynette has relied on hoʻoponopono, a respected practice that emphasizes the healthy relationships of family members. She is one of a handful of kūpuna who practices and teaches hoʻoponopono today. Pukui, Haertig, and Lee (1972) state that hoʻoponopono occurs in a "specific family conference in which relationships are set right through prayer, discussion, confession, repentance, and mutual restitution and forgiveness" (60). Pule is fundamental to hoʻoponopono.

Living and Learning Hawaiian Culture

Having descended from a lineage of healers on her mother's side, Lynette's exposure to Hawaiian healing practices began at a very young age (DeMattos 2016). "Because I was reared with my grandparents, I was able to observe and learn pule ʻohana [family prayers], and at that time, nobody could go to sleep at night if there was pilikia [trouble, distress]. My mother came from a family of ten, so we always had hoʻoponopono," said Lynette.

She explained that the differences in personalities among siblings often can lead to differences in opinions, which can lead to dissent. In her family, such differences and dissent were reconciled with prayer. For Lynette, the most important way to bring healing and healing practices back to Hawaiian families is through the consistent observation of pule ʻohana (family prayers).

These prayers linked Hawaiian families to Hawaiian gods or to the Christian God and were always a major part of the prevention of or remedy for discord (Pukui, Haertig, and Lee 1972).

Lynette's father was a man of few words and did not share much of his mo'okū'auhau with her other than to tell her that he was a "pure Hawaiian man from Hālawa, Moloka'i." Lynette was in the sixth grade, eleven years old going on twelve, when she told her father that she wanted to learn about her Hawaiian family. From that moment on, Lynette spent all of her summers with her father's 'ohana on Moloka'i. She says, "I got to learn the Hawaiian way of living, and it was survival." Lynette fondly recalls spending time with her sister and their cousins, nieces, and nephews catching 'o'opu (freshwater fish) in the streams, gathering limu kala on the shores, and pounding kalo into poi for every meal. "The time I spent on Moloka'i helped me to see that I was Hawaiian, and this is how we live," she said.

There was no running water in their home on Moloka'i. Once water was brought to the house, she said, "we washed everything, including our clothes, by hand. We hung everything on lines to dry, which came with lessons meant to teach us kids to kilo [closely observe]." She went on to explain that the hana (work) was not pau when the clothes were hung. It was also their kuleana to make sure that, if rain came, the clothes would not get wet. This meant that they had to use their observational skills to identify weather changes and take quick action if necessary.

There was no electricity in the home. There was "no radio," she said. "You had to entertain yourself! So I played 'ukulele." For Lynette, entertaining herself, and others, came easily. For as long as she can remember, she and her father would have weekly jam sessions: "After we pau eat [finished eating], if I saw him going to get his 'ukulele, I'd go get mine, and we'd sing together." Having been raised attending church at Kawaiaha'o, Lynette learned hymnal songs that enhanced her ability to pick up music faster than most: "I can hear the song and make the harmonic changes, because my ear is naturally attuned to the chords. My cousins and I would sing four-part harmonies together from the sixth grade on." Later in life, Lynette played and sang with Leo Nahenahe, a four-piece group that also included Noelani Kanoho Mahoe, Mona Akiona Teves, and Ethelynne Soares Teves. These four wāhine played Hawaiian music together for more than forty years, performing mele of old Hawai'i they learned from their kūpuna.

A significant part of Hawaiian pedagogy is observation, a practice that Lynette is very familiar with. As a child, she learned to observe the environment. This strengthened her connection to the ʻāina. Lynette also learned to observe familial and cultural practices, which strengthened her connection to ʻohana and community. These observations were both formal, such as pule ʻohana, and informal, such as food preparation. The synthesis of these experiences created a strong kahua (foundation) from which to learn, practice, grow, and eventually teach.

O KE KAHUA MAMUA, MAHOPE KE KŪKULU.

The site first, and then the building.

(PUKUI 1983, 268)

This ʻōlelo noʻeau reminds us that a firmly set kahua, including connection to one's land, family, and community, encourages the perpetuation of the principles, practices, and protocol of the ancestors.

Grounding in Social Work and Hoʻoponopono

Lynette began attending the Kamehameha Schools in Kapālama, Oʻahu, in the seventh grade. The school offered a "Christian education," which, as she states, "offset the type of education" she'd been exposed to until then and opened her up to opportunities that would shape her future. Lynette worked hard to find a balance between a childhood of Hawaiian cultural values and the practices of a Christian education that emphasized Western ways. In pursuit of balance, Lynette remained paʻa (firm) in her self-identity and steadily and consistently worked toward pono behavior.

Seeking balance for herself also meant helping others to find that balance, and Lynette began to realize early on that she wanted to help others. She recalls an English assignment she received in her freshman year at Kamehameha Schools. The task was to write a paper on a potential career path. She said, "I did my research, and what do you know, my paper was about social work," a profession dedicated to helping others.

After high school, Lynette set her sights on Bradley University in Peoria, Illinois, where she completed two years before returning home to complete her bachelor's degree in sociology. She then applied and was accepted to the University of Hawaiʻi at Mānoa (UHM) School of Social Work's master's program. It is here that she met Richard Likeke Paglinawan, who received his degree in June 1962. Likeke and Lynette married that September. After learning she was pregnant with twins, Lynette decided to focus on her growing family. She returned to the university in 1964 and attained her master's in social work in 1966. She was the only Native Hawaiian in the program at that time. The dominant social work pedagogy of the 1960s, according to Lynette, "was all Western theory." As Western as it was, Lynette discovered that social work, with its focus on helping others, strengthened her self-identity as a Hawaiian woman.

After receiving her master's in 1966, Lynette accepted a position from the Queen Liliʻuokalani Children's Center (QLCC). The leadership at QLCC had a vision that would require the expertise of individuals who understood the value and significance of Hawaiian culture relative to Western theories and practices of social work.

Likeke was already working at QLCC when Lynette joined the staff. Lynette remembers a time when Likeke worked closely with a Hawaiian family who had cultural difficulties that could not be resolved with social work rooted in Western theories and skills. He shared this with Myron "Pinky" Thompson, the executive director of QLCC at the time. A social worker of Hawaiian ancestry, Pinky understood the value, importance, and need of perpetuating Hawaiian ideologies, especially those that involved healing, health, and wellness. Thus, the QLCC Cultural Committee was established in 1965 with the following members: Betty A. Rocha, MSW, ACSW (chairman); William Apaka Jr., MSW, ACSW; Marian C. Haertig, MA; Grace C. Oness, MSW, ACSW; and Richard "Likeke" Paglinawan, MSW, ACSW.

The primary purpose of the QLCC Culture Committee was to rediscover the Hawaiian practices of the ancestors that have relevance for Hawaiian familial relationship issues in contemporary times (Paglinawan and Paglinawan 2012). Under the guidance and tutelage of Mary Kawena Pukui, a highly distinguished Hawaiian expert, the QLCC Culture Committee provided guidance and support for the seminal texts *Nānā I Ke Kumu* (Look to the Source) volumes 1 and 2. Both volumes have cultural knowledge that provides "bridges to an understanding of our ancestors viewed from our present complex system of thinking, feeling and doing" (Pukui et al. 1979, v). These books contain information for effectively working with Hawaiian families. An important practice highlighted in the books was hoʻoponopono.

In 1969, Lynette was asked by QLCC to be the lead research practitioner for a project whose goal was to provide hoʻoponopono to families. Her task was to assess each family for its fit with hoʻoponopono and to document the process. As a social worker, Lynette worked with families to address social issues. As an educator, she taught families the process of hoʻoponopono to restore and empower their own family functioning. She felt that it was important to train a member of each family in hoʻoponopono, stating, "If I could train at least one family member to be the healer, everyone would now have access." The research and data derived from this study set standards for the teaching and practice of hoʻoponopono, and helped to prevent the practice from being exploited or watered down through misuse. The outcome of this study, she said, set the direction that "hoʻoponopono is viable with Hawaiians today and, in fact, is transferrable."

Hoʻoponopono—Background and Context

In old Hawaiʻi, Hawaiians lived in isolation for generations upon generations. They developed complex systems to address all types of situations for the individual, family, and community in the context of the environment and spiritual realms. They also understood, accepted, and lived knowing the importance and value of relationships. If there was pilikia, it was best to address issues quickly and efficiently to prevent further discord. However, restoration of ʻohana relationships can be complicated, as noted in this ʻōlelo noʻeau:

HE NAHĀ IPU AUANEʻI O PAʻA I KA HUPAU HUMU.

*It isn't a break in a gourd container that can be
easily mended by sewing the parts together.*

(PUKUI 1983, 91)

Hoʻoponopono was practiced in traditional Hawaiian communities to help resolve conflict within the ʻohana.

Upon the arrival of Christianity in Hawaiʻi, many traditional practices were forced underground or ceased to exist. Hoʻoponopono, once a foundational family healing practice, became devalued and demonized. Because some components of hoʻoponopono were thought to appeal to "pagan gods," hoʻoponopono practice was labeled as pagan (Pukui, Haertig, and Lee 1972). Some Hawaiians came to believe that their time-honored method of family therapy was a "stupid, heathen thing," and, like many other cultural traditions, its practice began to deteriorate.

"History may fade, rituals may be discarded, and customs changed with the passage of time. Yet many of the basic values of Hawai'i's past remain vital and true and applicable in the present day" (Pukui, Haertig, Lee, and McDermott 1979, xi). Despite societal changes, ho'oponopono, like other cultural practices, such as lua, lā'au lapa'au, and lomilomi, endured and remained vital to Hawaiian culture.

With dedication to the perpetuation of ho'oponopono, Lynette, along with Likeke, advanced its development for and application to Hawaiian families in need. They refined the definition and description of "ho'oponopono": "A process of prayer, self-scrutiny, insightful confession, repentance, mutual restitution, and forgiveness between involved parties in consort with the powers they believe in. The process of ho'oponopono addresses several levels at once: the cognitive level, which is about information gathering, the level of interpersonal relationships . . . then [we go] to a deeper level . . . to get at underlying issues that often prevent people from fully moving on" (Paglinawan and Paglinawan 2012, 14).

Ho'oponopono is an 'ohana practice, and as such, variations exist. However, several fundamentals are common components of the practice. Lynette shared the essential attitudes, purpose, and procedures of ho'oponopono as it was taught to her by Mary Kawena Pukui (Paglinawan and Paglinawan 1991). For example, ho'oponopono can be used in the diagnosis, remediation, or prevention of conflict. An essential attitude is 'oia'i'o (truth, sincerity). Participants must agree that problems be discussed one by one and that they are self-scrutinizing and willing to control disruptive emotions by channeling discussion through the leader. They must use explicit and specific communication, provide answers in the positive, and not withhold secrets. They must accept that the leader may call for periods of calm to facilitate control of tempers and self-inquiry or to allow participants to rest during an all-day session. The essential procedures include:

* Pule wehe (opening prayer). The leader provides an opening prayer that asks the powers that be for help, wisdom, understanding, and sincerity.
* Kūkulu kumuhana (statement of the problem). In this phase, there is agreement on the statement of the problem and procedures for seeking solutions. It calls for the pooling of emotional and spiritual forces through prayer, and acknowledges that the ho'oponopono leader will reach out to resistive participants.

* Wehena (period of discussion). In this phase, there is a discussion with three key elements.
    * Mahiki (handling one problem at a time). Each person talks with the leader, one by one, about the incident, taking into account each person's feelings and reactions. The leader handles one problem at a time, from its beginning, setting it to right. As in the peeling of an onion, mahiki is the disposing of one layer of action, motivation, or emotion at a time.
    * Hihia (the entanglement of emotions, reactions, and interactions all in a negative way through acts of commission or omission) and hala (transgression). Recognition of entanglements and transgressions on both sides—one bound by the fault one has committed, the other by holding on to the injury.
    * Hoʻomalu (to make calm or to provide a period of silence). Hoʻomalu is declared when the family members need to "cool off," to think things over, and to refrain from any other activities.
* Mihi (to repent and forgive). As participants gradually understand the situation through the identification of the hala and the hihia, the next step is mihi, in which they repent and forgive. Forgiving means to forgive fully and completely and without reservations. Forgiveness is sought and given for each specific problem and is not generalized. Where restitution is necessary, it is arranged for and made.
* Kala each other completely. This is a mutual process wherein the wrongdoer and the wronged are released from each other. It means "I unbind you from the wrong and thus may I also be unbound from it."
* ʻOki. In this phase, the ties to the problem are severed in the physical, mental, and emotional sense. When ʻoki is genuine, kala becomes possible. The ʻoki severs and separates the wrongs, the hurts, and the conflicts so the negative effects are removed and participants feel a deep sense of resolution.
* Pule hoʻopau (closing prayer). This prayer provides a summary of what has been resolved and an affirmation of positive individual and ʻohana functioning.
* Pani (closing ritual). This usually involves the offering of food to the powers that be and acts of purification and prayer. A pani is done at the termination of the entire treatment process or when a big problem has been resolved.
* Na hana imua (future tasks). Once the family sets to right the conflict, they then identify new goals and prepare to implement them.

Pukui, Haertig, and Lee (1972) state,

> Hoʻoponopono seems to be a supreme effort at self-help on a responsible, adult level. It also has the spiritual dimension so vital to the Hawaiian people. And even here, prayers, to aumakua in the past or God in the present, are responsible, adult prayers. The appeal is not the child-like, 'Rescue me! Get me out of this scrape.' Instead it is, 'Please provide the spiritual strength we need to work on this problem. Help us to help ourselves.' Hoʻoponopono may well be one of the soundest methods to restore and maintain good family relationships that any society has ever devised. (69–70)

The potential for healing is great, but so too is the responsibility: "When you do hoʻoponopono, it is a great responsibility, kuleana; you deal with [people's] lives on a much deeper level. If you're not careful, you can make mistakes and injure people. You could also injure yourself and your family" (Paglinawan and Paglinawan 2012, 22).

Hana (Work) and Legacy of Hoʻoponopono

Since leading the 1969 hoʻoponopono project, Lynette has accepted and embraced her kuleana as a Native Hawaiian social worker who draws primarily from Hawaiian practices. She has since touched the lives of thousands of families and haumāna through hoʻoponopono. The deep-seated love she holds for her people, her culture, and the lāhui is what fuels her passion for continuing this very significant work.

An important part of Lynette's kuleana has been teaching. Lynette was an instructor and curriculum developer at Windward Community College from 1977 to 1978, and she was a practice methods instructor for the bachelor of social work (BSW) and master of social work (MSW) programs at the Myron B. Thompson School of Social Work at the UHM from 1978 to 1981. In 2005 and from 2008 to 2017, Lynette reengaged in teaching activities at the school, served as a cultural consultant for various school initiatives, and directed the Hawaiian Learning Program (HLP) (DeMattos 2016). The first cohort of HLP (1975–1980), under the direction of June Oda, graduated approximately forty Native Hawaiian MSWs with a deep understanding of Hawaiian approaches to social work practice. From 2008 to 2017, Lynette, Likeke, and ʻAnakē Malina Kaulukukui ran the HLP, sharing Hawaiian knowledge and social work approaches with approximately seventy-five

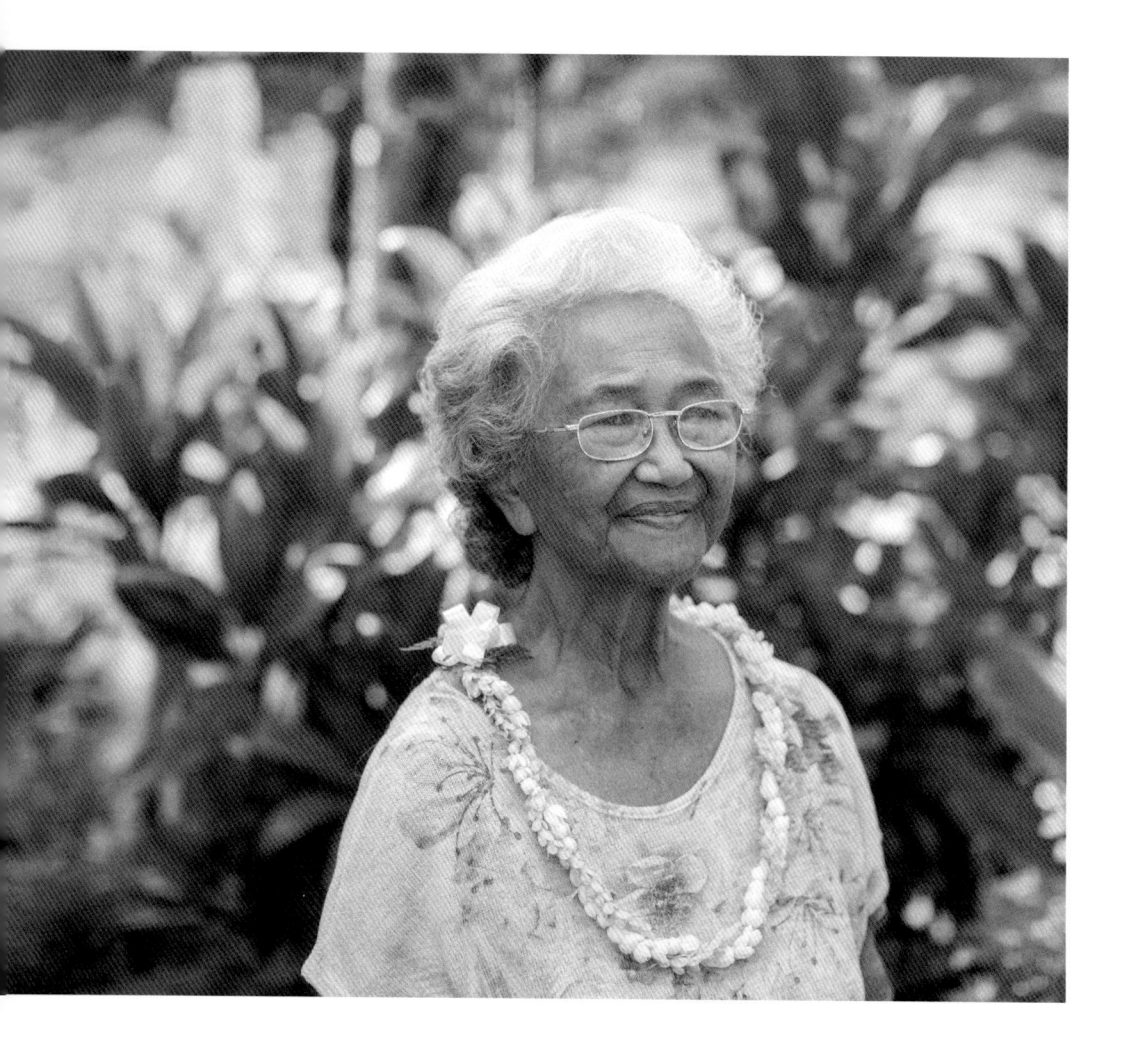

Native Hawaiian MSWs (Mokuau 2019). Starting in 2017, Lynette moved to University of Hawaiʻi–West Oʻahu to work with Hale Kuahuokalā, where students entering the health field are taught about traditional practices to provide more effective health care in Native Hawaiian communities (Avendaño 2019). Many have acknowledged ʻAnakē Lynette for her love of Hawaiian music and culture, and her selfless dedication and commitment to the betterment of the Hawaiian people.

Over the last few decades, ʻAnakē Lynette has been recognized by countless organizations and associations. For example, in 2010, she received the Native Hawaiian Education Association's Educator of the Year Award.

Also in 2010, she and her husband Likeke received the Institute on Violence, Abuse, and Trauma Award for the promotion of Hawaiian culture. In 2011, she and Likeke were honored with the Kaonohi Award by Papa Ola Lōkahi. In 2012, she was honored with the I Ulu I Ke Kumu Award by the University of Hawai'i at Mānoa Hawai'inuiākea School of Hawaiian Knowledge.

To perpetuate Hawaiian culture, "you have to train students for service toward future generations . . . if not, then our traditions will not be perpetuated" (Paglinawan and Paglinawan 2012, 14). Lynette has seen the power of transferability firsthand. Her vision of teaching and empowering families to reclaim their health, healing, and well-being for themselves is steadily coming to fruition. She continues to strive to restore healers to every Hawaiian family, and says, "I envision a time when families nurture their relationships, mālama or care for each other, and deal with problems while they're simple and uncomplicated."

Lynette and Likeke are known for their lifelong dedication to teaching and practicing cultural ways. In 2020, along with coauthors Dennis Kauahi and Valli Kalei Kanuha, they continued the legacy of the Nānā I Ke Kumu with the production of a third volume (Paglinawan et al. 2020). This volume "strives to expand the teachings of Mary Kawena Pukui" and emphasizes historical trauma, kaumaha (grief), and ho'oponopono. Lynette and Likeke often share these words of wisdom with family, friends, and haumāna: "With the loss of culture goes the loss of identity. With the recovery of culture is the recovery of identity. Self-esteem and confidence can grow. And with those, perhaps Hawaiians can deal better with today's society."

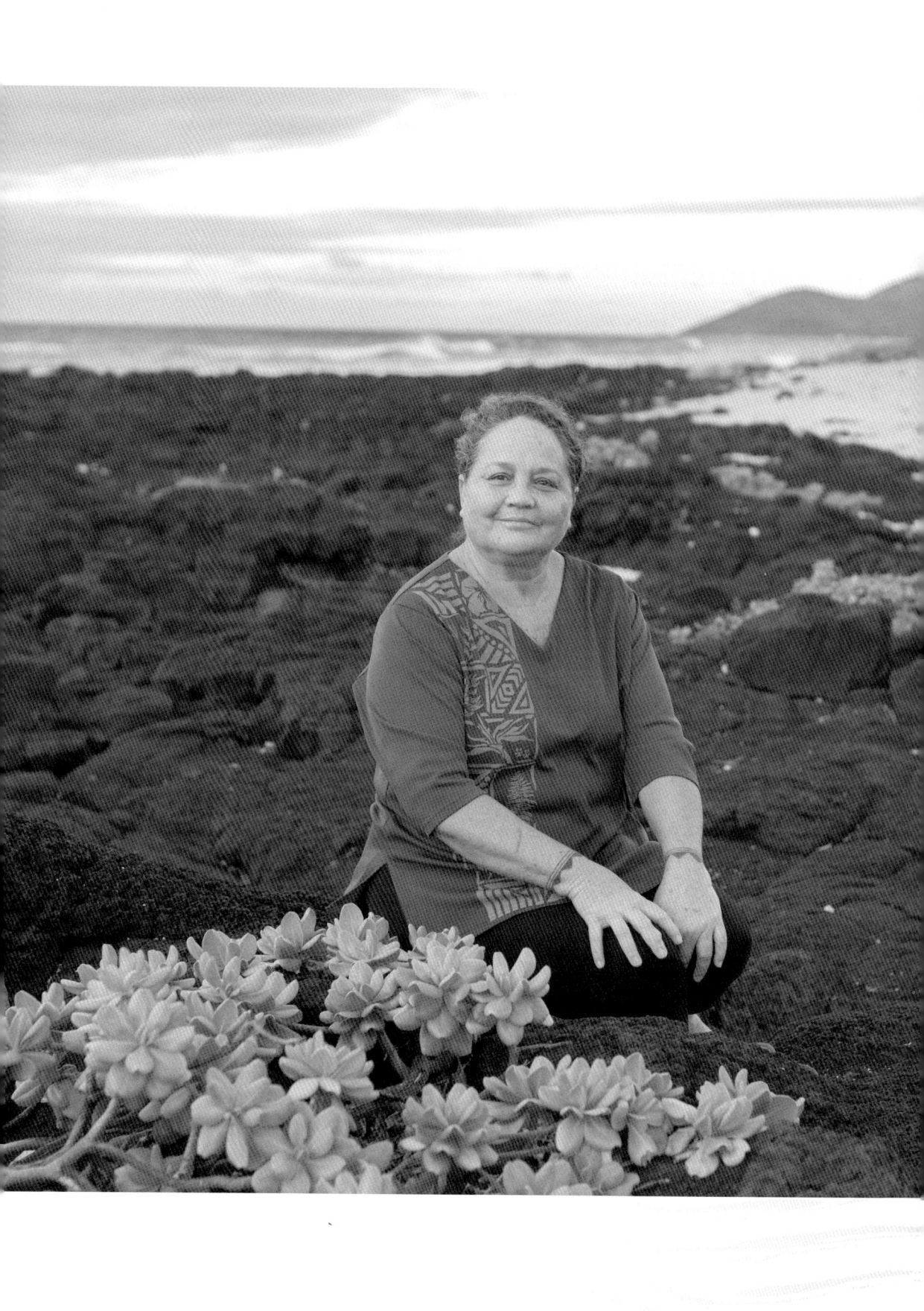

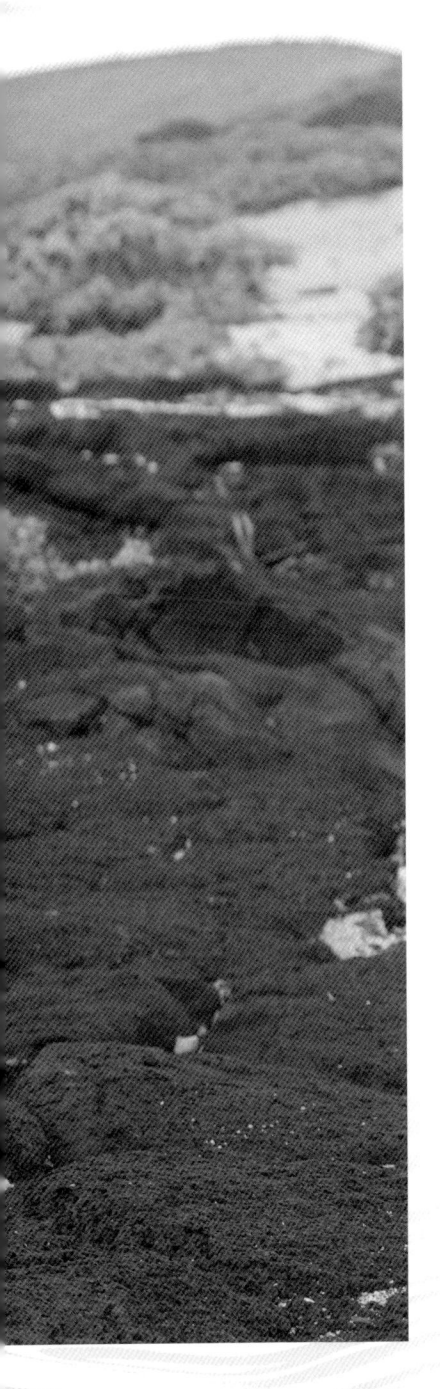

CHAPTER 9

Sharon Leina'ala Bright

LĀʻAU LAPAʻAU

Sharon Leina'ala Bright is a practitioner of lāʻau lapaʻau, a Hawaiian healing practice using Hawaiian medicinal plants (Abbott 1992). She integrates this healing practice with lomilomi and pule and works alongside Western medicine practitioners as a traditional healer at the Waimānalo Health Center on Oʻahu. She believes that the integration of healing approaches can help advance health equity and social justice in Hawaiʻi.

An Integrated Beginning

Leinaʻalaʻs life reflects an integration of backgrounds and approaches. She was given her first name Sharon by her Irish mother, and her middle name Leinaʻala by her Hawaiian father. In starting our meeting, she offered a pule beginning with "Na Iehova Ke Akua e alakaʻi me ke aloha" (with the loving guidance of our Heavenly Father). She then chanted her moʻokūʻauhau back eight generations. In sharing her prayer and her koʻihonua (genealogical chant), she says, "I am calling on Ke Akua, ʻaumākua, and my family to bring wisdom, spirituality, and sacredness to our conversation and practice."

‘O kēia ka moʻokūʻauhau o ka ʻohana Bright
‘O Keōua ke kāne
‘O Kekuʻiapoiwa ka wahine.
Noho pū lāua, a hānau ʻia ʻo Kamehameha.
‘O Kamehameha ke kāne
‘O Kanekapolei ka wahine
Noho pū lāua, a hānau ʻia ʻo Kahiwa Kanekapolei.
‘O Namiki ke kāne
‘O Kahiwa Kanekapolei ka wahine
Noho pū lāua, a hānau ʻia ʻo Puahaunapuako.
‘O Ewaliko Piʻimauna ke kāne
‘O Puahaunapuako ka wahine
Noho pū lāua, a hānau ʻia ʻo Hanamuahaleonaihe.
‘O Andrew Nohokaikaleikini ke kāne
‘O Hanamuahaleonaihe ka wahine
Noho pū lāua, a hānau ʻia ʻo Andrew laukea Kelii Kinaihai.
‘O Andrew laukea Kelii Kinaihai ke kāne
‘O Alice Keahi Kao o Pololu Kekipi ka wahine
Noho pū lāua, a hānau ʻia ʻo Solomon Kamaluhia Kekipi Bright.
‘O Solomon Kamaluhia Kekipi Bright ke kāne
‘O Wanda Bernice Rogers ka wahine
Noho pū lāua, a hānau ʻia ʻo Victor Kaleoaloha Kealii Kaapuni Houston Bright.
‘O Victor Kaleoaloha Kealii Kaapuni Houston Bright ke kāne
‘O Frances LaVerne Chism ka wahine
Noho pū lāua, a hānauʻia ʻo Sharon Leinaʻala Bright
‘O wau ʻo Sharon Leinaʻala Bright.
E ola ka Hāloa o koʻu ʻohana Bright. E ola!
Mahalo. Mahalo. Mahalo.

Leina‘ala's family is originally from North Kohala on Hawai‘i Island, and the Brights descend from one of the Kamehameha lines. In the mid-1800s, one of Leina‘ala's ancestors, John Kekipi Maia, became a leader of a religion called Hoʻomana Naʻauao, based on a philosophy of "reasonable service" as presented in Romans (12:1) in the Bible. This religion has been described as a blend of Christian and Hawaiian faith. Maia traveled around the islands preaching his message and was granted land on Oʻahu to build a church, called Ke Alaula O ka Malamalama. "This church, also known as Bright's Church, was built in 1897 on Cooke Street in Kakaʻako, and our family home was next to it," says Leinaʻala. "My father was the last in our line to be born in that house." The church, rebuilt in the late 1960s, still stands today amid the tall buildings of Kakaʻako.

Leinaʻala's grandfather, Solomon Kamaluhia Kekipi Bright, was an entertainer who worked for a time in San Francisco, along with Hilo Hattie and others. "At the Fairmont Hotel," she said, "he oversaw five different ballrooms and Hawaiian entertainment. They even built a raft to float in the Fairmont swimming pool, carrying a Hawaiian band and hula dancers to entertain the guests." Her grandmother, Wanda Bernice Rogers, was part Hawaiian and part Katzie First Nation, an Indigenous tribe in British Columbia. Wanda was the descendant of a Native Hawaiian fisherman, Kimo Keamo, who settled in Western Canada and married a local Katzie woman (Koppel 1995). Wanda had moved to California to act in movies that needed to cast Hawaiian and American Indian characters, and there she met Sol Bright. "My grandparents met in California, and the love story started from there," said Leinaʻala.

Leinaʻala was born and spent her first eighteen years in the Bay Area before moving to Hawaiʻi. "But our lifestyle in California was very Hawaiian," she says. "My family steeped us in our culture, the moʻolelo, the values, the music, the food." Leinaʻala remembers that prayer was a big part of daily life and healing within the family. Leinaʻala's mother was a nurse who used home remedies and provided most of the family's primary and preventive care. "I was a little different from the rest of the family," remembers Leinaʻala. "I would go off and spend time in the mountains and bring home plants and animals. I was always curious in those realms." Leinaʻala felt a connectedness to the spiritual and to healing, and when she was very young she would pray to become a healer. Given her ancestral ties to healers and ministers, her desire to become a healer was not surprising.

Integrating Hawaiian Healing Practices

Leinaʻala is a practitioner of lāʻau lapaʻau. Using prayer as a foundation, she integrates lāʻau lapaʻau with lomilomi. These three practices are traditionally intertwined. She says, "If you look at the moʻokūʻauhau of lāʻau lapaʻau, it leads you back to the order of Lonopūhā (first student of Kamakanuiʻahaʻilono, god of healing). If you look at lomilomi, it leads you back to the order of Lonopūhā. Prayer is essential to both, and it links us to the highest source." She notes that some people, like kumu Levon Ohai, practice only lāʻau lapa'au, and some people practice only lomilomi. But many people practice both, including Auntie Margaret Machado. "She applied lomilomi, lā'au lapa'au, and prayer in a ten-day course of cleansing, and look how powerful her healing work was," says Leina'ala.

Leina'ala's training in the healing arts began at home, learning from her mother and father. When she moved to Hawai'i in the 1980s, she studied lomilomi with kumu Alva Andrews. Kumu Andrews' technique involves massage and realignment and can be traced back five hundred years through the Pe'a 'ohana lineage on the island of Hawai'i. In July 2000, Kumu Andrews and Leina'ala started their own lomilomi practice in Waimānalo. The name of the practice, Ka Pā Ola Hawai'i, was given to them by Dr. Ishmael W. Stagner, kumu hula and professor of education, psychology, and Hawaiian studies. In the 2000s, Leina'ala studied lā'au lapa'au with kahuna Levon Ohai.

In addition to training in lomilomi and lā'au lapa'au, Leina'ala strengthened her cultural learning in other practices, including hula from renowned kumu hula Kaha'i Topolinski of Ka Pā Hula Hawai'i and lua from 'Ōlohe lua Mitchell Eli and Jerry Walker of Pā Ku'i-a-Holo. The intense training required in these various approaches and Leina'ala's thoughtful integration of them supported her overall practice in the healing arts.

From her lineage in the Pacific Northwest, she learned about the Northwest Coast people's healing practices and heard the prayers of her great-grandmother in her native Katzie language. Leina'ala experienced the Si.Si.Wiss medicine teachings and healing ceremonies through Johnny Moses, a Tulalip Native American master storyteller, oral historian, healer, and spiritual leader: "Storytelling, laughter, song, drumming, and other healing methods are used in Si.Si.Wiss medicine. I feel fortunate I was able to experience this powerful medicine."

Although different practitioners embrace different styles according to their teachers, families, and ahupua'a, Leina'ala recognizes that spirituality, nature, and prayer are foundational to all the practices and that they are interlinked. "Through the practice of lua, I learned to link my breath, mana, and prayer for a deeper form of healing. Through lua and hula, I learned to draw on the masculine and feminine energies exemplified by Kū [Hawaiian God] and Hina [Hawaiian God]." Being skilled in multiple interrelated practices expands one's ability to assess, diagnose, and call on different tools to address the needs of the person who has come for healing.

Practicing both lomilomi and lā'au lapa'au allows Leina'ala to draw on her knowledge of lā'au (plant, medicine) to make her own oils for lomilomi, as well as her own poultices, teas, tinctures, and salves for healing. She maintains lā'au gardens at her home and workplace, the Waimānalo Health Center. She calls her gardens Ka Waihona Lā'au Lapa'au, which translates to "the herbal medicine cabinet." She gives an example of her integrated practice: "If you come for lomilomi, I might also prepare you a tea or a poultice to continue your healing. And then the prayer continues all the time, before and after you have made contact, and from that point on."

Learning Lā'au Lapa'au

Leina'ala began her training in lā'au lapa'au within the Waimānalo community and through her studies at Windward Community College and the Hawai'inuiākea School of Hawaiian Knowledge at the University of Hawai'i at Mānoa. At Mānoa, she studied with kahuna Levon Ohai, whose history and philosophy were documented by his student kumu Keoki Kīkaha Pai Baclayon. Levon Ohai learned lā'au lapa'au from his grandfather, Benjamin Ohai, who learned from his parents, Kekauaimokuohaikainoa and Akio Aki. Although traditional protocol would not have supported the teaching of Hawaiian healing arts through university settings, Kahuna Ohai believed it was important to expand the number of lā'au lapa'au practitioners so that every home could have a healer. His vision was to develop practitioners that were strong in spirit, had respect for protocol, and were diligent in procedural compliance and willing to become perpetual students of the practice (Baclayon 2012).

Kahuna Ohai taught about the healing power of plants and prayer. He also taught about the role of the lā'au lapa'au practitioner in the prevention of disease, stressing the importance of addressing lifestyle, and not just treating (and perhaps masking) symptoms. Thus, he stressed the importance of the seven laws of ola (health), which include a good diet, adequate sleep, regular exercise, cleansing, meditation, pondering, and pule. He also taught his students that practitioners should speak softly and kindly, no matter what the situation, and should not judge. Kahuna Ohai considered multiple factors in selecting certain plants to be used as remedies, including patient factors, the season, moon and ocean cycles, the characteristics and maturity of the plant, and the plant's growing conditions (Baclayon 2012). He also stressed the importance of mālama 'āina.

Leina'ala remembers how Kahuna Ohai would describe a plant and tell students to collect it for the next class. In following his teachings, she would search for a makua (adult) plant, say prayers, and ask permission from the plant before collecting. She looks for the strongest plant to gather, as noted in this ʻōlelo noʻeau:

NĀNĀ NO A KA LĀʻAU KU HOʻOKĀHI.

Look for the plant that stands alone.

(PUKUI 1983, 248)

In class, Leinaʻala noticed that many students initially made errors and picked the wrong plant or picked too many plants from the same place. Worried that students and others would start to strip accessible areas of the forest, Leinaʻala started her lāʻau gardens to conserve Hawaiʻi's natural areas. "I would look near the makua plant for baby plants," she said. "If I was told through prayer that a keiki plant would be willing to go with me for the purposes of medicine and teaching, I would bring it home." Keiki plants willing to be transplanted survived well in her aquaponics system, which combines hydroponics (soilless horticulture) and aquaculture (raising fish in tanks), recycling the waste from fish into the water used to nourish plant growth (Ho-Lastimosa et al. 2019). "This is an excellent environment to start the keiki collected from the forests, because it is so rich," she says. Not all lāʻau lapaʻau practitioners would consider growing plants for medicinal use, instead preferring to collect them in the wild, but Leinaʻala is committed to preservation and conservation, as well as healing. She adds, "Some varieties of plants are never willing to come home with me, so these varieties I still gather, following traditional protocol."

The Waimānalo aquaponics project is operated by the University of Hawaiʻi College of Tropical Agriculture and Human Resources, and this group helped Leinaʻala set up her home aquaponics equipment. Leinaʻala is a firm believer in aquaponics, and a teacher of using aquaponics to grow lāʻau. She explains, "Expanding aquaponics to every Hawaiian household in Waimānalo is helping us gain food sovereignty. Using aquaponics to grow lāʻau will help with medical sovereignty too. We can be self-sustainable within our community."

Both native and introduced lāʻau can be cultivated in one's yard, māla (garden), or aquaponics system. Leinaʻala uses and teaches her patients to use ʻawapuhi (ginger), nīoi (Hawaiian chili pepper), ʻōlena (turmeric), ōwī (blue vervain), comfrey, laukahi (plantain), noni (Indian mulberry), pohekula (Asiatic pennywort), pōpolo (glossy nightshade), pōhinahina (sedge), kālika (garlic), and other plants. As Kahuna Ohai reminded his students, plants used for lāʻau lapaʻau are warriors, each with unique skills and characteristics to fight illnesses (Baclayon 2012). He often quoted an ʻōlelo noʻeau that refers to the ʻaʻaliʻi (native hardwood shrub), which can stand the worst of winds, twisting and bending but seldom breaking or falling over:

HE ʻAʻALIʻI KU MAKANI MAI AU;
ʻAʻOHE MAKANI NANA E KULAʻI.

I am a wind resisting ʻaʻaliʻi;
no gale can push me over.

(PUKUI 1983, 60)

Integrating Traditional and Western Care

In 2015, Dr. Mary Oneha, the Waimānalo Health Center director, invited Leinaʻala to help the center integrate traditional and Western care. Leinaʻala spent her first year introducing staff to lāʻau lapaʻau so they would understand the practice and how it could complement Western care. Training included the health center's physicians, who have been open-minded about the mission of integrating various approaches to healing, believing in the need to be open to healing in its many forms. Leinaʻala says, "Because of busy schedules, time constraints, and insurance reimbursement, physicians try to keep their clinical exams to twenty minutes. In the beginning, I was just bridging that gap with the doctors. I can talk with patients like a friend, like an auntie, like a younger sister, to ask them. ʻSo, what's going on? Why are you here today? How can I help you, Auntie?'"

Now, as one of the health center's Native healing practitioners, Leinaʻala works beside a primary care provider. "The doctor likes that we meet with the patient together. While she's talking to them, I can work on shoulders and arms and help relax the patient and improve the quality of health care interaction." Together, the practitioners can look at multiple aspects of a patient's health—physical, mental, emotional, and spiritual. The goal is to look at health and well-being from the patient's perspective and use a team of providers to holistically assess and help the patient. Patients have more options and can decide when it's more appropriate to use one type of care over another. In many cases, the teas, salves, and poultices from lā'au lapa'au have worked better than Western medicine, especially for skin ailments. For example, a patient with a cyst was told by the doctor that it needed to be lanced, which would leave a scar. Instead, Leina'ala tried a lā'au poultice, and the cyst resolved in two to three days without scarring. Because of these options, patients are more enthusiastic about coming to the health center. Seeing the esteem in which traditional healing approaches are held at the health center has brought another dimension into their lives and has helped them to balance their Hawaiian traditional beliefs with Western beliefs (Spencer and Oneha 2019).

Leina'ala also helps her patients master the seven ola laws pertaining to diet, sleep, exercise, cleansing, meditation, pondering, and pule. For example, the Waimānalo Health Center team includes a nutritionist to help patients make better diet decisions. Leina'ala teaches patients to prepare their own lā'au lapa'au and promotes aquaponics to increase patients' access to healthy foods and medicinal plants. Behavioral health providers and counselors help with emotional and mental health. Pule promotes spiritual as well as physical health. Leina'ala believes that without changing one's lifestyle to honor the seven ola laws, taking lā'au will only treat the symptoms, not the underlying causes of ill health: "You must be willing to make changes. If I just hand you lā'au and we do not offer the prayers or do the work that goes along with it, then you just have plants without the spiritual power to heal. We must remember the link between 'āina, the practitioner, and Ke Akua is prayer. The healer is the conduit."

Teaching Lā'au Lapa'au

Long before foreigners began to arrive in Hawai'i, Native Hawaiians had already developed a highly organized, locally based health system. The healing traditions included training in the cultivation, gathering, and preparation of lā'au, lomilomi, ho'ohāpai (induction of pregnancy) and ho'ohanau keiki (baby delivery), 'ō'ō (bloodletting), hāhā (palpation), ha'iha'i iwi (bone setting), 'ike lihilihi (close observation), and the calling and engaging of spiritual forces (Abbott 1992; Malo 1951).

For many centuries, the closeness between Kānaka and the 'āina provided an opportunity for careful research to understand and venerate local

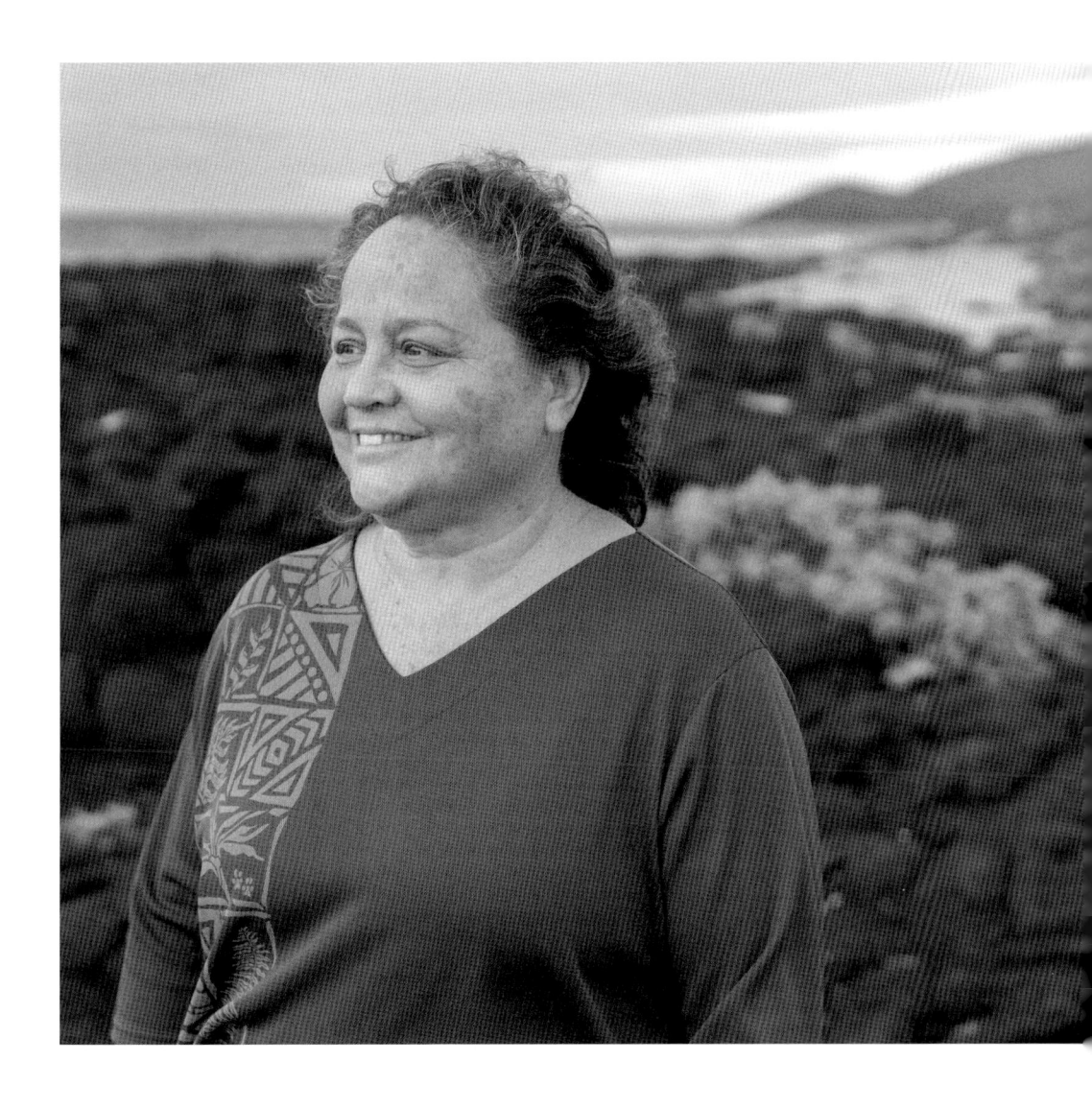

plants and learn about their specific effects on the human body (Mitchell 2001). The effects varied, depending on where the lā'au was grown, when it was gathered, how it was gathered, who it was gathered by, and its age. "In some prescriptions, a part of one plant, such as the bud or bark, would be the only medicine prescribed. For other treatments, the medicine would be compounded from two or three or even ten or more herbs" (234). Uses of lā'au and other elements in the environment were effective because of their spiritual and metaphorical mana (Handy and Pukui 1972).

Traditional healing practices were discouraged by missionaries who arrived in Hawai'i in the early 1800s, by legislative acts in the 1860s, and following the illegal overthrow of the Hawaiian Kingdom by the United States in 1898. In 1911, a law was passed that lā'au lapa'au practitioners, referred to by the Hawaiian Medicine Board as "herbalists," had to be licensed. Two of the three board members were Caucasian, and they instituted a certifying examination that required applicants to know and use the Latin names for native medicinal plants. As a result, few lā'au lapa'au practitioners applied for or were granted licenses (Donlin 2010). "The lā'au lapa'au practitioners went underground," says Leina'ala.

The Hawaiian Renaissance of the 1970s started to bring more attention to the link between poor Hawaiian health and the colonization of the Hawaiian nation. In 1978, the state sponsored a constitutional convention, and several constitutional amendments to redress the loss of land and culture were proposed and passed by the Hawai'i State Legislature. One amendment guaranteed Hawaiians access to the mountains and the sea in support of Hawaiian hunting and gathering traditions, including the gathering of lā'au. In 1988, the federal government passed the Native Hawaiian Health Care Improvement Act, which recognized and defined Native Hawaiian traditional healers as those whose "knowledge, skills, and experience are based on a demonstrated learning . . . acquired by direct practical association with Native Hawaiian elders and oral traditions" (Native Hawaiian Health Care Improvement Act 1988). In addition to the Waimānalo Health Center, the Wai'anae Coast Comprehensive Health Center, the Waikiki Health Center, and the Native Hawaiian Health Care Systems on each island offer patients access to traditional healing practitioners.

As in the past, established practitioners of lā'au lapa'au are teaching the next generation. One of the best-known teachers of lā'au lapa'au in the past thirty years was Papa Henry Auwae, who initiated hundreds of haumāna across the state into the practice (Auwae 2000). Besides traditional healers themselves, some information on lā'au lapa'au is being gleaned from the large collection of Hawaiian-language nūpepa now digitally archived on the Ulukau Hawaiian Electronic Library.

In addition, courses in lā'au lapa'au are offered on several campuses in the University of Hawai'i system. Kahuna Levon Ohai was the first teacher of this practice on the Mānoa campus, and kumu Keoki Baclayon filled this role upon the passing of Kahuna Ohai in 2012. Keoki also works with patients at the Waimānalo Health Center. Together, Keoki and Leina'ala offer a three-year certificate program called Papa ʻĒwekea Piʻi Moʻo Lāʻau Lapaʻau, funded by a grant from the US Administration for Native Americans through Sustain Hawaiʻi, a nonprofit in Waimānalo. The first year focuses on past wisdom of the ancestors, including their use of meditation, prayer, oli, listening, and discerning, as well as protocols in gathering, preparing, and using lāʻau. The second year focuses on the "now," examining the intimate relationship among Ke Akua, ʻaumākua, people, and the environment and integrating practices that move students to know what it really means to "make things right" through the connection and unity of all elements. The third year focuses on the future, including the kuleana of being a practitioner on all levels—spiritual, mental, emotional, and physical. Haumāna learn in the classroom and field and complete preceptorships at Waimānalo Health Center, shadowing Leinaʻala and Keoki.

Although Leinaʻala is a teacher of lāʻau lapaʻau, she also recognizes her role as a haumāna (student) and is excited about the reawakening of Hawaiian knowledge. She says,

> One of my quests at the health center is to role model how we can learn together. As I teach, I remind participants that I am haumāna too and I'm here to help us to remember what our families did to heal ourselves. For example, once I was demonstrating the use of ʻuhaloa [small, downy American weed], an important lāʻau for your garden. You can make a tea from the inner bark of the root. It is good for sore throat, as it's highly antiinflammatory. A woman shared that her grandmother infused ʻuhaloa into a steam bath for a woman who has just given birth. This helped to shrink the skin and uterus back to normal size and to heal perineal lacerations. It was such a great piece of information for us all to learn. So part of my work is to perpetuate the knowledge by reawakening it in others. We can now openly remember and talk about our traditional practices and help make sure they get passed down.

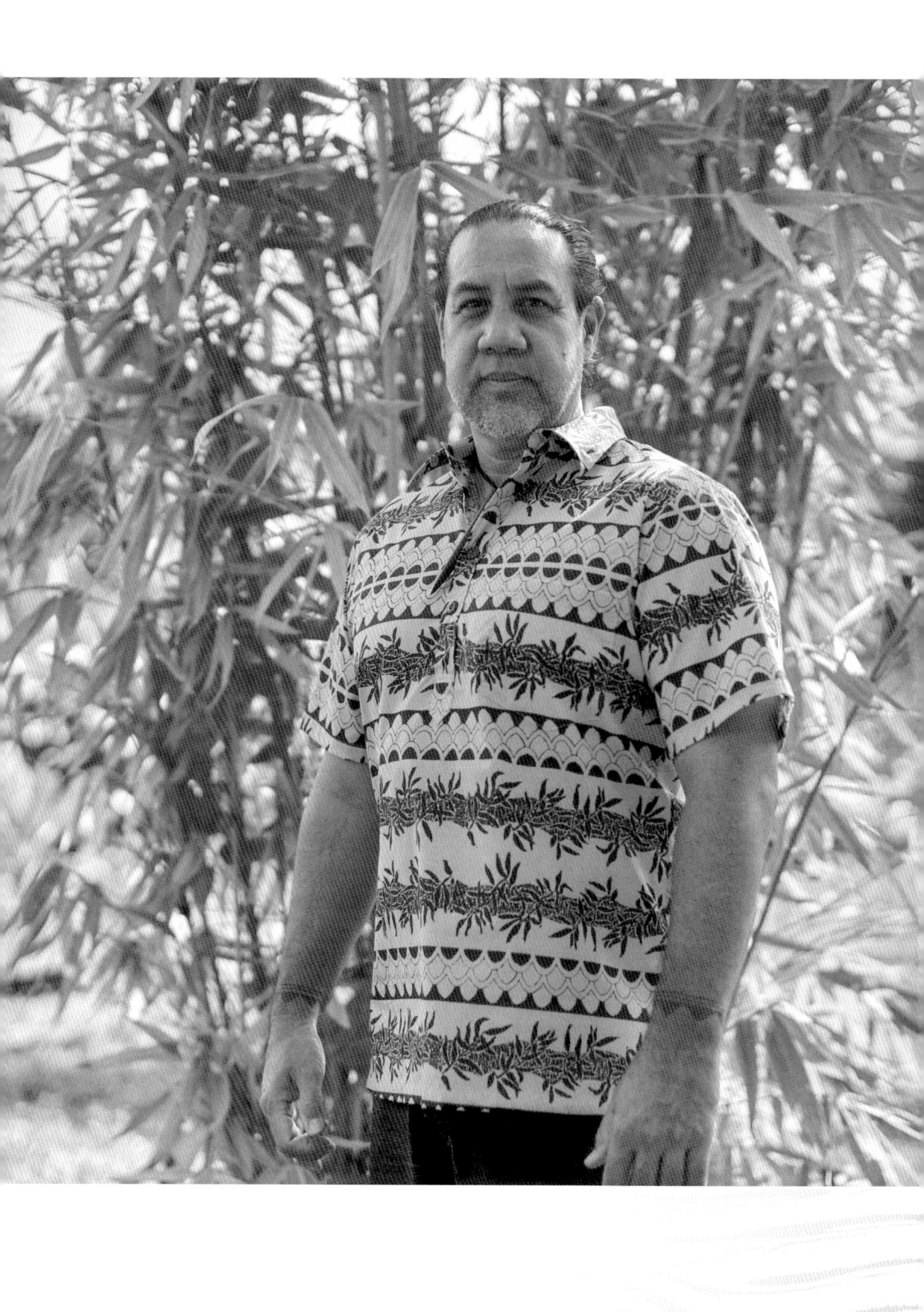

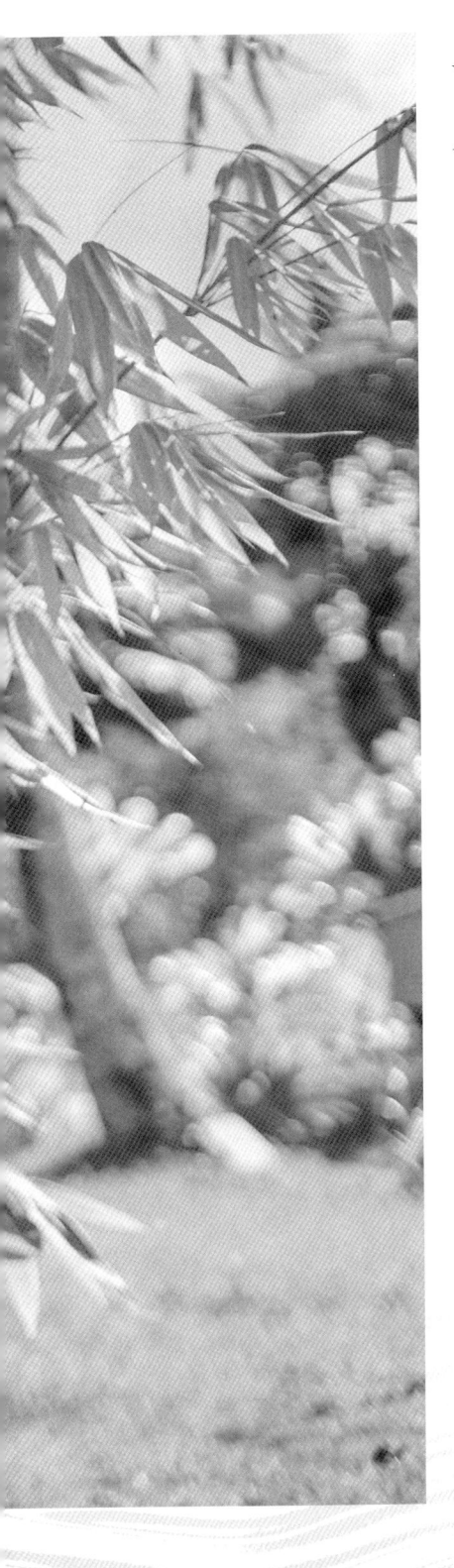

CHAPTER 10

Keola Kawaiʻulaʻiliahi Chan

LOMILOMI

Keola Kawaiʻulaʻiliahi Chan relies on ʻike kūpuna (ancestral knowledge) to learn about the healing practices of traditional Hawaiʻi. Of the twenty-three healing practices in the health system of traditional Hawaiʻi (Fox 2017), Kumu Chan is one of a few people today who has deep knowledge and training in multiple specialties, including lomilomi, hoʻoponopono, lāʻau lapaʻau, lāʻau kāhea (a type of faith healing), hula, oli, and ʻai kūpele (therapeutic nutrition). Of these, perhaps he is best known as a master healer and teacher of lomilomi, the practice to rub, press, knead, and massage.

ʻIke Kūpuna as a Basis for Healing Practices

The path to becoming a highly regarded healer of lomilomi was circuitous. Keola recognizes this when he says, "At first, it wasn't something that I actively chose." The combination of life experiences, personal attributes, and ancestral guidance eventually led Keola to healing. "Up until the late 19th century, the [Native] Hawaiian view of disease, medicine, and the body was intertwined with the indigenous notions of the self and with

Hawaiian cosmology" (Inglis 2005, 226). For Keola, his development as a healer might be viewed in the context of the natural environment and Hawaiian cosmology, with specific reference to the moon.

Keola's journey in the healing arts and as a master healer is eloquently framed by three significant, sequential phases of the moon: huna, mōhalu, and hua (phases eleven, twelve, and thirteen). The documented characteristics of these three moon phases and Keola's path to becoming a healer share similar implications of inquiry, discovery, exploration, acceptance, and perpetuation. The traditional Hawaiian lunar month cycles through thirty moon phases (Polynesian Voyaging Society n.d.), which are divided into three anahulu (a period of ten days). The first ten-day period is called hoʻonui, meaning "to enlarge" (Kamakau 1976). The second is called poepoe, "round." And the last anahulu is called hoʻēmi, "to diminish." Each month starts with the new moon, hilo, waxing through ten phases (hoʻonui), rounding through ten phases (poepoe), waning through ten phases (hoʻēmi), and ending with muku (last moon of the thirty-day moon cycle). Maintaining a connection to the moon and the environment helps to reestablish and affix to ancestral knowledge, which informs us in a variety of ways about the present and the future.

Huna is the eleventh moon and appears in the anahulu poepoe period. According to Pukui and Elbert (1986), a huna is a minute particle, a grain, a speck, a minutia, something small or little. "Huna" also means "hidden secret" or "hidden." Huna represents the inquisitive younger years of Keola's life when he focused on and excelled notably in music and when lomilomi remained hidden from his consciousness.

Mōhalu is the twelfth moon and also resides in the period of anahulu poepoe. According to Pukui and Elbert (1986), "mōhalu" means "to open or unfold like a flower." Mōhalu represents the time in Keola's life when, as a middle-aged adult, he discovered and began to explore his interest in the healing arts of traditional Hawaiʻi. He sought guidance and teaching from renowned practitioners in various specialties. As his gifts in lomilomi and other healing practices unfolded, he was encouraged by his teachers to be open to the possibility of becoming a healer.

Hua is the thirteenth moon, and "hua" means "fruit" or "fruitful." Hua represents the present and future period of Keola's life, a period in which he has accepted his kuleana as a healer and has collaboratively developed a number of health-related initiatives. As his visibility and reputation in the community as a master lomilomi healer grew, Keola focused on developing methods to strengthen and institutionalize the practice. Along with colleagues, he established three nonprofit groups dedicated to healing. These groups are Hui Mauli Ola, ʻAha Kāne, and Ka Pā o Lonopūhā.

"It's taken time for me to understand what lomilomi was, what it's become, and that the health needs and remedial preferences of Hawaiians are diverse," says Keola. He continues, "Sometimes traditional approaches are preferred, sometimes Western ones, and often a blend of both. We need traditional healing practices to get to a point where they are presented as viable options or alternatives to patients, among Western ones. I believe we must provide the most informed, highest-quality, patient-centered treatment plan to meet the diverse needs of Hawaiians. To do so, we must accept and offer various treatment preferences, which include Hawaiian, contemporary, and a blend of both."

Lomilomi as a Healing Practice

Wellness is often viewed as the healthy functioning of an individual in balance in relationships with the family, community, environment, and spiritual realm. This balance can be expressed through the idea of dualism, a concept that permeates all aspects of Native Hawaiian culture. In their cosmology, Native Hawaiians recognized the dualism of complementary opposites such as sky and earth, sun and moon, day and night, male and female, spiritual and material, health and illness, and life and death (Blaisdell 1997). Dualism provides a foundation for a holistic understanding of the natural environment and demonstrates the relationships between the biotic and abiotic world. Its function is to conceptualize and help maintain balance. The balance between health and illness relies heavily upon observation, evaluation, and diagnosis. When an individual becomes ill, it is believed that there is a source of imbalance. Fox (2017) states that kūpuna are able to diagnose the true source of the imbalance and recommend treatment strategies accordingly. Treatment strategies vary and often include some form of lomilomi.

Lomi means "to rub, press, squeeze, crush, mash, knead, massage, and rub out" (Pukui and Elbert 1986). When the term "lomi" is repeated, as in "lomilomi," it represents a stronger emphasis of meaning. In old Hawaiʻi, Hawaiians knew herbal remedies and how to massage: "Parents and grandparents used lomilomi to mold the features of children and make them strong. In turn, children were trained to lomi adults . . . and were often seen treading on [them]. Adults in the family [also] gave lomilomi to each other" (Chai 2005, 25).

Lomilomi was part of regular daily lifestyle, but it was also part of the complex health care system in traditional Hawaiʻi that required years of training (Fox 2017). In a traditional healing practice, Keola notes that it is important to do an assessment or diagnosis before treatment. He states, "We must look at the order. Before you lomilomi, you have to be able to assess and diagnose your client properly to provide treatment options that facilitate the best possible outcomes, and realize that sometimes it doesn't require lomilomi." According to Keola, there are four quadrants of wellness that every healer considers when performing diagnoses. These are the physical quadrant, which is the most visible, and the spiritual, mental, and emotional quadrants, which Keola refers to as the unseen areas. "When sickness or illness manifests into the physical realm," he says, "it has more than likely already had adverse effects on the three unseen areas—spiritual, mental, and emotional. The skill of the healer lies in the curtained spaces."

Lomilomi, along with the other healing arts of traditional Hawaiʻi, had a place in supporting and maintaining the health of Native Hawaiians. The healer could alleviate joint pain, set bones, calm muscle spasms, strengthen connective tissue, and reduce tension and swelling, and would often use various oils and ointments to reduce inflammation, as well as to rejuvenate the skin and the epithelial tissue, muscles, and nerves (Fox 2017). Throughout the book *Nā Moʻolelo Lomilomi,* practitioner, author, and teacher Makana R. Chai (2005) describes lomilomi in relationship to other traditional Hawaiian medicinal and health practices: "Traditional practitioners documented a wealth of information about lomilomi as medical therapy. Native healers used lomilomi massage with hāhā, lāʻau lapaʻau, wai ola (water and heat therapies), haʻihaʻi iwi, hahano (cleansing), and ʻōʻō to remedy specific diseases. It is only lomilomi as restorative massage that was rarely documented by native historians" (34–35).

There are legendary moʻolelo that attribute the genealogy of the healing arts to Lonopūhā (Crabbe et al. 2011). Lonopūhā was an aliʻi who gave up his chiefly status after being cured by Kamakanuiʻāhaʻilono, a healer who decided to leave the realm of the gods to help humankind counter the spread of sickness and disease set forth by other deities such as Kaalaenui-ahina, Kahuilaokalani, and Kaneikaulanaula (Thrum 1907). The healing skills and powers of Lonopūhā became so great that his status was eventually elevated. Lonopūhā set a clear path that paved the way for the development and perpetuation of healing practices taught to him by Kamakanuiʻāhaʻilono and others.

Keola states, "What we learn through moʻolelo is how we should conduct ourselves as kumu, haumāna, and, most importantly, as healers. It also provides an opportunity for us to reflect on who we are, what we do, and where we need to go."

Huna

While there are elements of Keola's childhood and young adult life that provided subtle hints that foretold the kuleana in the healing practices he'd come to know, like the characteristics of the huna moon, most of it remained hidden from his consciousness. Keola grew up in Papakōlea, a Hawaiian homestead in urban Honolulu on the island of Oʻahu, surrounded by an ʻohana of healers, mostly of Western practices, including nurses, doctors, and emergency medical technicians. Keola states, "Even though I was around and exposed to different Western healing practices, I don't remember ever really being into healing. It wasn't a path that I actively chose." Although Papakōlea is where his roots remain, Keola, like many Hawaiians, maintains deep connections to other places across the pae ʻāina (archipelago). These places include Kahaluʻu and Kawaihāpai Waialua on Oʻahu and Pukuilua in East Maui.

For Keola, life events and personal attributes served as precursors to becoming a healer. This is similar to traditional times when kāhuna in the healing arts were chosen based on genealogy, the outward and inward purity of the healer, and the healer's piety (Hewett et al. 2001). Keola believes that his destiny as a healer may have been set even before his birth. He recalls his mother telling him that doctors informed her that she would be unable to conceive children. The unexpected birth of Keola convinced her that having a child improved her health and was a healing experience. "Growing up, my mom was constantly telling me that story. I must have heard it a hundred times," Keola states. "I will always remember her saying that having a child helped her heal."

Keola always found substance in the oral traditions of his ancestors, and he perpetuated these oral traditions through music. He learned from many highly honored and respected musicians, including Ainsley Keliʻi Halemanu, George Holokai, Kimo Alama Keaulana, Kahauanu Lake, and Kaʻupena Wong. Playing Hawaiian music provided Keola with a strong cultural foundation embedded in Native Hawaiian practices, protocols, and beliefs. He used this foundation in educating children and adults in the art of music compilation, translation, arrangement, and instrumentation.

Performing and teaching music were life events that may have served as precursors to Keola's life as a healer. Music has healing properties, as it can ease anxiety and discomfort during procedures, restore lost speech, reduce the side effects of cancer therapy, aid in pain relief, and improve the quality of life of people with dementia (Harvard Health 2016).

As his musical talents were being fostered and developed, Keola began to experience situations that prompted and reinforced his interest in health and healing. "I remember it like it was yesterday," he begins. "One night, I was on a break from playing music at a gig when a woman approached me from behind, grabbed my hand, and began to study my palm with intent."

"You're going to do lomilomi," she proclaimed.

"Okay, auntie," Keola replied. "Mahalo for the insight."

He never saw that woman again. Around the same time, Keola was preparing to have his first child, and, not knowing how to be a father, a sense of panic set in. He felt an urgency to "figure it out," as he states. One day while walking around Windward Mall in Kāneʻohe, Keola passed what was then called the Lomi Shop. A woman came out of the shop, approached him, and asked if he'd like to work there. "I don't even know what you do here," Keola says as he began to look up at the name of the shop. "The Lomi Shop?" he says. He instantly remembered the encounter with the woman who studied his hands and spoke prophetically about his becoming a lomilomi practitioner. Keola took full advantage of his schedule as an evening performing musician and spent his days at the Lomi Shop, observing the client / practitioner interactions and relationships. Keola noted the mutual respect and reverence given and received by both client and practitioner and immediately knew that this was something special and something he wanted to be a part of.

Mōhalu

As the twelfth moon phase, mōhalu, so vividly describes, the flower slowly unfurls its petals, and metaphorically, so does Keola's interest in seeking out traditional healing knowledge and practices. Having spent a significant amount of time at the Lomi Shop, Keola learned that the kūpuna were the modern-day keepers of lomi knowledge. Kūpuna in every ʻohana helped to transmit the knowledge of lomilomi for uses in daily life, but extensive knowledge and training were the materials for building lomilomi as a specialty in the healing arts. Keola remembers, "One day, I was talking with my grandmother about the lady who read my palm and how it led me to the Lomi Shop. . . . She told me she knew a renowned kupuna and teacher of lomilomi, Auntie Margaret Machado." She and Auntie Margaret had been school classmates. She also said that my uncle trained with Auntie Margaret some time ago. Unfortunately, by the time Keola's grandmother called Auntie Margaret, she was no longer teaching lomilomi. However, she had a student, Sheila O'Malley, that had permission to teach Auntie Margaret's work. Sheila had taken Auntie Margaret's advanced coursework and assisted her in her classes. "I never got around to calling her," Keola states. "Some time had passed when Sheila's name came up again, and I was encouraged by other individuals to contact her. So this time I did." This step was a benchmark in formal training in lomilomi and grounded Keola in roles of healer and advocate for traditional healing arts.

After completing training with Sheila, and with her encouragement, Keola went on to pursue the teachings of renowned hoʻoponopono practitioner Auntie Malia Craver. After completing his training with Auntie Malia, Keola went under the tutelage of lāʻau lapaʻau practitioner Auntie Alapaʻi Kahuʻena. After many years of training under various expert practitioners, Keola began to notice slight differences in their practices. "I started to notice that, directly or indirectly, practitioners began making assumptions that their way was the best way." But because Keola had taken classes from so many different practitioners, he held a unique perspective that one approach or style may be suitable for one type of person or ailment but not for others.

Hua

Hua, the thirteenth moon phase, describes the present time in Keola's life where there is a convergence of experiences from conception, childhood, and early adulthood with his training in ʻike kūpuna from noted kumu. For Keola, the merging of knowledge from life experiences and rigorous training in the healing arts bears the fruits of achievement and leadership in lomilomi and other healing arts. In addition to being a healer, Keola has invested his life in the perpetuation of ancestral knowledge through the establishment of three nonprofit organizations, Hui Mauli Ola, ʻAha Kāne, and Ka Pā o Lonopūhā. While these organizations differ subtly in purpose and scope, they commonly focus on the health and well-being of Native Hawaiian communities, the perpetuation of the healing arts for present and future generations,

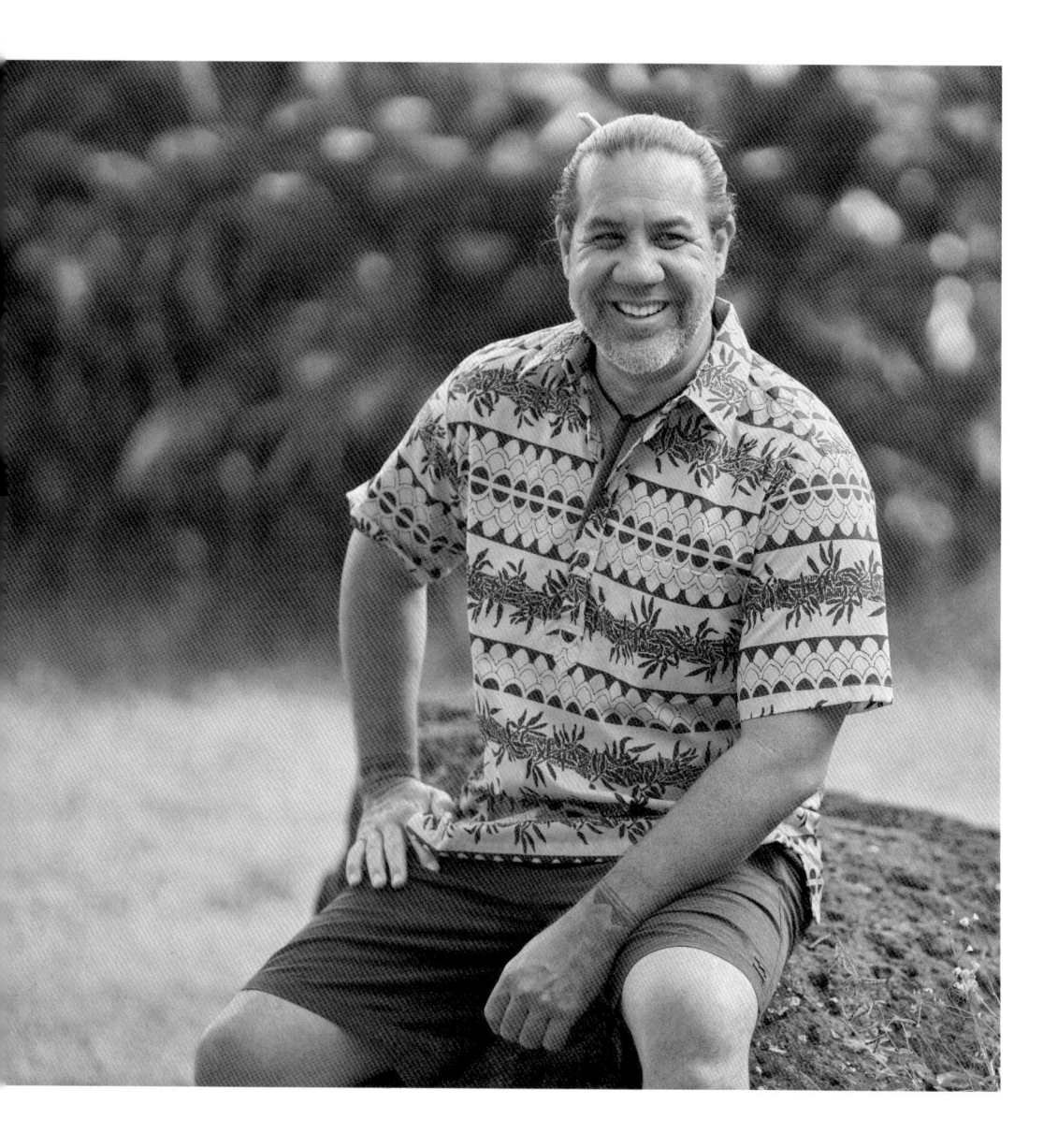

and kuleana healing art practitioners and kāne for healthy families and communities. Hui Mauli Ola was founded in 2006 and is rooted in Hawaiian traditions and spiritual practices. Its primary purpose is to create spaces where kūpuna can share traditional healing practices with the younger generation of upcoming practitioners. It is an organization of multidisciplinary cultural practitioners committed to promoting and improving the health and well-being of our communities through empowering and providing access to quality care and educational opportunities. Its purpose is to

1. Support intercultural exchange for practitioners to foster Indigenous healing knowledge;

2. Support the practitioner's development by creating interactive programs based on culture and land;

3. Support and develop multidisciplinary educational experiences for communities that encourage them to live healthy and productive lives;

4. Develop materials and programs to educate communities on Indigenous health practices;

5. Create environments for our traditional healing arts to thrive;

6. Protect the rights of traditional cultural practitioners; and

7. Promote the use of traditional healing practices.

Since 2013, Keola has taken the role of executive director of a nonprofit called 'Aha Kāne. 'Aha Kāne was founded by three of Keola's revered mentors: Dr. Kamana'opono Crabbe, 'Ōlohe 'Umi Kai, and 'Ōlohe Billy Richards. Its mission is to strengthen the Native Hawaiian community through nurturing and perpetuating traditional male roles and responsibilities that contribute to the physical, mental, spiritual, and social well-being of Native Hawaiian men and their families and communities ('Aha Kāne n.d.). Its vision is to nurture a healthier Native Hawaiian male population by eliminating psychosocial, health, and educational disparities through activities founded on traditional cultural practices that build sustainability in the community. In his work with 'Aha Kāne, Keola continues to make strides in increasing the health and well-being of Native Hawaiian men.

Ka Pā o Lonopūhā formed in 2010. The goal of this organization is to raise the consciousness of traditional Hawaiian healing and to revive the practice of lomi 'a'e, which is to massage the back with the feet. Ka Pā o Lonopūhā participates in various community events, including one held in September of 2019 at the Bernice Pauahi Bishop Museum through its Living Culture series titled "Hawaiian Health and Well-Being." The Living Culture series provides an opportunity for participants to meet Hawaiian practitioners, observe them as they practice their skill, and "talk-story" with them about their area of expertise.

Reflecting on the progress made and future work in reestablishing Hawaiian healing arts after decades of their suppression, Keola states,

> We're pretty good at treatment. Our kūpuna held on to that piece pretty well. We have to work backward to rebuild the other pieces, such as the diagnosis and assessment components. If Lonopūhā set a path to establish the practice of assessment and diagnosis at one time, it can be done again. We must be honest with ourselves and acknowledge the areas within our practice that we "forgot." It's not "lost." It's still there for us to restore, and it is up to us to rebuild the missing pieces. What will be the methodology? What is the process? And how are we going to get it done? This is all about kūkulu hou [rebuilding]. All we need to do is go back, identify and learn the missing pieces, and rebuild.

Healing as Service

Keola credits ʻike kūpuna for the healing practices of old Hawaiʻi and acknowledges that the perpetuation of healing as a service must originate with our kūpuna and our families. For Keola, learning can start with one's own family, with this set of questions: Who were the healers in your family? What were the sicknesses that you see replicated through time in your family? How far back, generationally, can you trace that sickness? What did your grandma cook for you when you were sick? What did your mom give you when you weren't feeling well? These are just a few questions that, according to Keola, "we must ask ourselves and begin documenting. It is where we must begin to reclaim autonomy of the health and well-being of ourselves, our family, and our community."

Keola reminds us that "healthcare and healers only exist because of the people they serve." Lomilomi exists to serve specific purposes but does not do so in isolation. There is a continuum of Hawaiian traditional healing practices for health promotion, disease prevention, and treatment. According to Keola, lomilomi "is low in the pecking order concerning the healing process and is only one of twenty-three known Native Hawaiian healing practices that reside within the traditional healthcare continuum." He continues, "Health is where we have to focus. We must begin to inspire our youth to get into healing. We must also look to the moʻolelo of our kūpuna, as they provide deep insight into our Hawaiian healing practices. Knowledge is ʻike, and ʻike is mana."

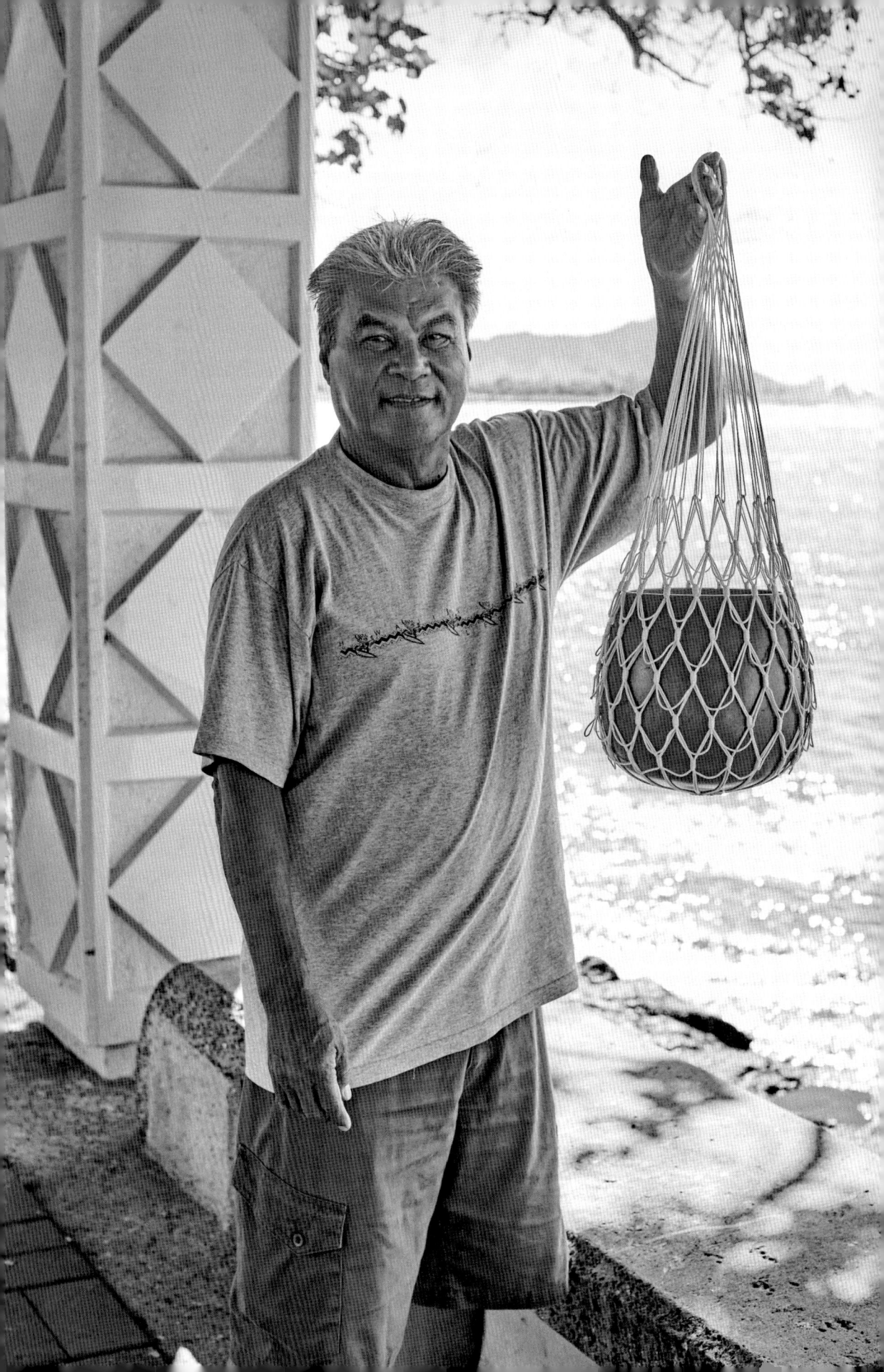

CHAPTER 11

Charles "Sonny" Kaulukukui III

KAULA

With a methodic rhythm, Sonny Kaulukukui demonstrates a practice of old Hawai'i called kaula—cordage and rope—as he sits erectly and uses his hands to gently roll, twist, and pull plant fibers. The making of kaula was a valued customary practice of old Hawai'i. One can almost imagine Hawaiian ancestors sitting under trees, enjoying a cooling breeze, and making kaula for articles of daily living, such as the netting to hold gourds containing water.

This practice has been adapted for use today. With a skillful repetition that has a hypnotic and almost meditative effect, Sonny twists plant fibers together to make a larger cord. With his left hand holding one end of the plant fibers, he rolls the fibers on his right thigh using the open palm of his right hand to twist them around each other to form a cord. This action repeats itself until the desired cord length and thickness are achieved. He is quick to note that "this is not the only way to do it, as kaula making may vary by training and purpose." It is easy to see that patience and stamina are required traits for the kaula maker, as the practice is exacting and time intensive. It is also possible to imagine the benefits of a tranquil calmness in this practice of Hawaiian ancestors.

Inspiration for Cultural Learning

Sonny did not learn kaula making from his family. Still, it is apparent that his "growing up years" provided the foundation that eventually inspired his pursuit and training in this practice. His mother's family was from Moloka'i, and his father's family was from Hilo, Hawai'i. His parents met in Kalihi, O'ahu, where Sonny's maternal grandfather worked at Kalihi Hospital, a detention and quarantine station for people with Hansen's disease. Sonny's grandfather took care of the buildings at the station, doing carpentry and other maintenance jobs.

Growing up in Kalihi, Sonny says that "my parents never really talked about culture, or maybe I missed it or wasn't ready to absorb it." But as he thoughtfully reconsiders and reflects on his past, he recognizes that his parents and extended family taught him the importance of culture through acts of everyday living. For Sonny, one way to absorb culture was by observing a senior family member. He recalls learning by observing and modeling behaviors shown by his uncle who lived next door. This ʻōlelo noʻeau is said of a careful observer like Sonny:

KA MANU KAʻUPU HĀLŌʻALE O KA MOANA.

The kaʻupu, the bird that observes the ocean.

(PUKUI 1983, 160)

In his early childhood Sonny would go shore fishing with his uncle at Sand Island, a small island at the entrance to Honolulu Harbor, Oʻahu. Fishing for food for the family included "informal" cultural instruction from his uncle, as Sonny learned about providing for the family, understanding natural phenomena such as ocean currents, and using fishing tools such as fishing rods and fishnets. It is interesting how early family education turns up in later life, as Sonny now practices kaula making, a tradition that created the fishnets in old Hawaiʻi.

As an adult, Sonny's interest in culture intensified when he started to learn and practice lua with Pā Kuʻi-a-Holo, a Hawaiian martial arts school. His early interest in lua developed because he thought "that lua was fighting and all that. I love doing that. But when I got into it, there was some fighting, but also history and learning about Hawaiian culture." With formidable leaders such as ʻŌlohe lua Mitchell Eli and ʻŌlohe lua Jerry Walker, Sonny learned that lua was more than just about fighting; it emphasized a way of life that held Hawaiian values and traditions as indisputable. Lua reinforced and complemented the more than fifty years of training that Sonny had in other martial arts disciplines. Sonny feels that constant practice was key to his learning.

E LAWE I KE AʻO A MĀLAMA, A E ʻOI MAU KA NAʻAUAO.

He who takes his teachings and applies them increases his knowledge.

(PUKUI 1983, 40)

With a steadfast commitment to lua, Sonny eventually achieved the elite status of ʻōlohe lua. Through his lua network, Sonny established lasting friendships and acquired knowledge and skills that would serve to move him deeper into his cultural heritage. It is not unusual to see Sonny with lua friends working on Hawaiian arts such as kaula and ʻohe kapala (bamboo stamps) at the Bishop Museum or toiling under the hot sun to preserve a wahi pana.

Sonny's inspiration for kaula making was circuitously linked to and reinforced by experiences in both childhood and adulthood. This type of grounding prepared him for a journey into learning a cultural craft that permeated every aspect of old Hawaiʻi.

Kaula as a Practice of Old Hawaiʻi

Sonny's interest and work in kaula was strengthened by a review of cultural works by distinguished Hawaiian historians such as David Malo and Samuel Kamakau, and supplemented by readings of botanical research by Catherine Summers. From these works, he learned about Hawaiian history, people's roles, plants, and cordage. Themes gleaned from his review of the literature are presented below.

In his learning from history books, Sonny knows that the value of cordage was best understood in context of the relationships of people, environment, and spirituality. In old Hawaiʻi, a thriving populace depended on a sustainable environment. People relied on natural resources for living and survival, and were vigilant stewards in caring for the land and ocean: "Cordage and rope of all sorts (nā kaula), were articles of great value, serviceable in all sorts of work" (Malo 1951, 78). Kaula was an essential component of daily life and requisite for constructing houses, building canoes, securing food with fishnets, and making tools such as adzes. Sonny says that one of his "go-to resources is the book *Hawaiian Cordage* by Catherine Summers who addresses the value of cordage." Summers (1990) states that "before the arrival of Captain Cook in 1778, the Hawaiians fastened things with cordage, for they had no nails, bolts, or screws" (1).

As with many things Hawaiian, tenets of spirituality in prayer and ritual undergirded the use of kaula. The consecration of a newly built house, the ritual for a new canoe, permission to use the adzes as tools, and the blessing of nets to catch fish were associated with nā pule kahiko (ancient Hawaiian prayers). A Hawaiian prayer speaks to the preparation and use of olonā (native shrub), a plant whose bark makes a strong fiber used to create fishing lines and nets:

Kuhi kuu ka lani   *I, as chief, willingly*

Keaweawekaokai honua,   *Cast my net of olona,*

Kupu ola ua ulu ke ipuu.   *The olona springs up, it grows,*

Ke kahi 'ke olona.   *It branches and is cut down.*

Kahoekukama kohi lani,   *The paddles of the chief beat the sea.*

(GUTMANIS 1983, 72)

The importance of the durability of the cord from which the fishnets were made is evident in a delightful tale of kaka uhu (fishing with a decoy fish). Fishermen, like farmers, carried the heavy responsibility of providing food for the people in the ahupua'a, and thus exercised great skill in the preparation of their tools and in the securing of food:

> The fisherman had his head underwater looking for fishes where he could spew forth chewed kukui meat into the sea. One hand directed the movements of the decoy uhu, and the other hand sculled the paddle to keep the nose of the canoe headed into the wind. When the fisherman saw a visitor uhu "kiss" the decoy uhu two or three times, he pulled the decoy uhu up, tilted the net into the sea, tied the decoy securely inside the net and lowered it down. When the net was properly placed with the decoy uhu, and the fisherman saw the visitor uhu come into the net and "sleep with" the decoy, he would pull the line of the net to entrap the uhu in it. (Kamakau 1976, 65)

Sonny is quick to note that there are numerous historical examples of cordage use in old Hawai'i. One example relates to the house that served as the primary shelter for the family, and thus had to be constructed with care and the best available materials. Cordage was used in the construction of houses to lash beams to wall posts and to lash rafters to beams. Homes were set on platforms of rocks, "where supporting posts are set firmly into the platform, and beams and rafters carved to fit at the joints are assembled with sennit lashings" (Kāne 1997, 62). In addition, furnishings such as "containers and water bottles made from gourds, some encased in basketry and hanging in netting from wooden racks," were displayed in homes (62). Once the work on the house was completed, it was customary for a prayer to be recited to consecrate the house before living in it.

Another example in which cordage was used relates to the adze or ax. This was a primary tool used for many tasks, including cutting trees for all types of woodwork. Perhaps one of the most important tasks for which the adze was used was canoe making. The adze was made of stone, wood, and string, and adze makers "were a greatly esteemed class in Hawaii" (Malo 1951, 51). Cord was braided and used to lash the handle to the axe. In the important work of canoe making, there were prayers said to "awaken" the adzes to begin the work: "The adzes were awakened by dipping them in the ocean as the kahuna called out 'E ala i hana no Kane' (Awake to work for Kane). They were dried and wrapped in tapa" (Gutmanis 1983, 75). After that, the workmen and kahuna would set out for the forest, carrying the adzes and other supplies, to secure the chosen tree. Cordage was also important in the transportation of the tree and the construction of the canoe. Once the tree was cut in the depths of the forest, "the bark of the hau tree [a type of hibiscus] was used for making lines or cables with which to haul canoes down from the mountains" to the ocean (Malo 1951, 78).

Learning from meritorious historians such as Malo and Kamakau provided Sonny with a formidable respect for history and culture. He imagined people doing what appears to be a simple task—making cordage—for significant outcomes such as the building of houses and canoes and the securing of food. This learning influenced his growth as a kaula maker.

Learning from Our History for Adaptation Today

The elemental use of kaula in all aspects of living in old Hawai'i made it important for all people to have some knowledge of and skill in kaula making. Sonny states that much of the learning was from within the family and the ahupua'a, and occurred through observation and modeling—as with a son imitating and learning from his father. In instances of specialized training, there was "instruction by experts. It was sound and excellent instruction, for it really was apprenticeship" in which a person might acquire a higher level of skill (Handy et al. 1965, 55). Sonny acknowledges that he received "specialized" training from renowned master weaver Patrick Horimoto. He says, "Patrick is known for his skillful weaving with the vine-like ʻieʻie [aerial roots] from the forest, and his creation of the authentically majestic mahiole [feather helmet]. As might be imagined with the apprenticeships of old Hawaiʻi, the teacher-student relationship between Patrick and Sonny is one of mutual respect. Their classroom is outdoors, near the ocean and under the shade of trees where both men work on individual projects. The student watches, sometimes asks questions, and then replicates. In words of praise, Patrick notes that Sonny attends to the detail required of kaula and has the skills of an artisan.

Sonny highlights three key areas for kaula making today: (a) materials for cordage, (b) cultivation and processing, and (c) techniques for cordage—twisting or braiding. His overview of these areas is informative and oftentimes laced with wistfulness and humor as he describes the adaptation of kaula practice for today. He talks about several materials used for cordage, including olonā and hau.

Olonā was a prized commodity in old Hawaiʻi because of the durability of cord made from its fibers. It was used in planting, fishing, and in other tasks in which binding and rope were necessary. The olonā bush is endemic to the Hawaiian Islands. Unfortunately, Sonny states that there is a relative absence of olonā today, likely because of challenges in its cultivation. He notes that the olonā is "really picky as to where they will grow, needing a lot of water, and perhaps even then, not thriving, because the water it needs would be that found in mists and sprays." There are few places where olonā will grow. It grows in rainy areas, in marshy places, and in those parts of the mountains that are always mossy from water and rain (Kamakau 1976). Although he is not aware of its cultivation today, Sonny reports that there may be some patches of olonā on the way to Hāna in Maui. He is wistful in his hope that someone from this or the next generation will have the resources to invest in cultivating this precious plant, which is integral to understanding Hawaiian history.

Hau was also valued and used widely for cordage in old Hawaiʻi, although it was not as water resistant or durable as olonā. It had sufficient strength to be used in thick cables or lines that would haul canoes down from the mountains, and it was also used for lashings for canoes and for netting to carry water gourds. It is believed to have been introduced by early

Polynesians, readily available in old Hawai'i, and thereby used broadly for daily living. Today, hau is still plentiful and grows abundantly on the lowlands and on the sides of the valleys.

While Sonny has experience in processing the raw materials for hau cordage, it is clear that it is not a job he relishes. In processing bark from the hau shrub, he states that you "have to locate the hau shrub, cut the branches, peel away both the inner and outer bark, immerse it in water, and scrape the gummy goo off the bark with hard pressure." He says that the scraping task is laborious work, often done on a board with a tool such as a shell to get the residue off. "This processing is important to prepare the fibers to get rid of the gummy stuff that bugs like in the bark," he says. It is arduous work. Sonny appreciates that Hawaiian ancestors devoted their time and energy to the processing and preparation of cordage, but laughing, and with a twinkle in his eye, admits that with modern advancements in cordage, he prefers to buy it rather than process and prepare it. His sources are Amazon, an e-commerce company, and a daughter-in-law and son who visit Japan frequently and willingly bring back ramie, a strong natural fiber of the nettle family.

Other materials used for cordage in the past and adapted for use today include the niu, which has fibers that can be twisted or braided into sennit for use with canoes or fishing; the hala (pandanus tree), which can be plaited and made into baskets and mats; and the ule hala (prop roots of the hala). Sonny says that you can create cordage from many other plants depending on your location, such as the koali (vine) that grows in the sand at the beach.

To create cordage, fibers were either twisted or braided. Twisting and braiding may seem straightforward, but they entail a meticulous level of detail and complexity by the artisans. Twisting a number of strands of fibers around each other to form a cord is called hilo (twisting). To make a strand, fibers are twisted in one direction, and to make a cord, two or more strands are twisted around each other in the opposite direction. Sonny makes cordage with skill and dexterity as he rolls, twists, and pulls strands across his right thigh. With the twisting style, Sonny creates the kōkō pu'upu'u (intricately woven netting) meant for a high-ranking person that will encase an ipu (gourd) or an 'umeke (bowl). The netting is a functional item that will carry the gourd or bowl, and it is also valued for its artistic beauty. Even with his level of skill, Sonny admits that it may take him three to four minutes to make one of the intricate knots on the kōkō pu'upu'u, and any error requires undoing the work and starting over.

With his background in lua, Sonny also creates weapons with cordage. One example is the leiomano (shark's teeth weapon), in which he uses lashings from abaca fibers from the banana trunk, which he forms with the twisting style, to hold the shark's teeth to the wood. The leiomano has the look of an oval hand mirror, and is a "hybrid between a shark-tooth club and a bludgeon dagger" (Hiroa 1957, 434). The durability and strength of the cords are important to this weapon of the warrior.

Braiding untwisted strands, typically three, to form a cord is called hili (braiding). Sonny says "it is like braiding a ponytail," where you start with three strands, and move the right strand over the middle strand, and then the right strand is now the middle strand, and the left strand must pass over it. With the braiding style, Sonny creates other Hawaiian weapons, such as the ka'ane (strangling cord), in which the braided cordage is attached to a wooden handle. Another weapon is the stone ma'a (sling), which has a pouch in the middle of two lengths of braided cordage. The ma'a was an important instrument used by the lua warrior: "First, the sling could be tucked in a malo during fighting, freeing both hands until it was needed. Also, the ammunition—unworked stones—could be found anywhere. All a warrior had to do was look on the ground" (Paglinawan et al. 2006, 51–52).

With both the ka'ane and the ma'a, an excess of the three-ply plait may be used to form stronger cordage, and this more difficult kind of braiding can cause complications. Sonny says that in complicated braiding, one may be working with eight strands, and thus you have "to pay close attention, because any error will cause you to hemo [untie] the entire process and start again." Sonny's Kumu Patrick is known to say, "Don't get lost, because it is hard to find your way back." The complexity of this craft increases the respect accorded to modern-day artisans and amplifies the preciousness of the final product.

Binding Our Generations

Sonny is animated as he teaches about kaula through "talk-story," demonstrates the techniques of twisting and braiding cordage, and displays cordage products. Kaula making has been a part of a larger life journey related to cultural learning and preservation. While Sonny is humble and unpretentious about his knowledge and skills, he is confident and emphatic about the value of this tradition for future generations.

He believes that his style of kaula making represents only one way of doing it, but that through this craft, we can preserve and perpetuate Hawaiian culture. Importantly, he thinks the perpetuation of the practice can contribute to cultural learning for students interested in social justice and health equity in two key ways. First, by reclaiming cultural traditions that were integral to life in old Hawai'i, he thinks that we can reduce the effects of cultural loss and trauma and reassert social justice. By understanding and practicing kaula, we are advancing the importance of the Hawaiian worldview linking people, environment, and spirituality, and perpetuating a valued and customary tradition. Second, he believes that engaging in the practice of kaula can lead to a cultural grounding and pride that builds esteem and identity, and ultimately, has restorative value in the health of Hawaiians and others today.

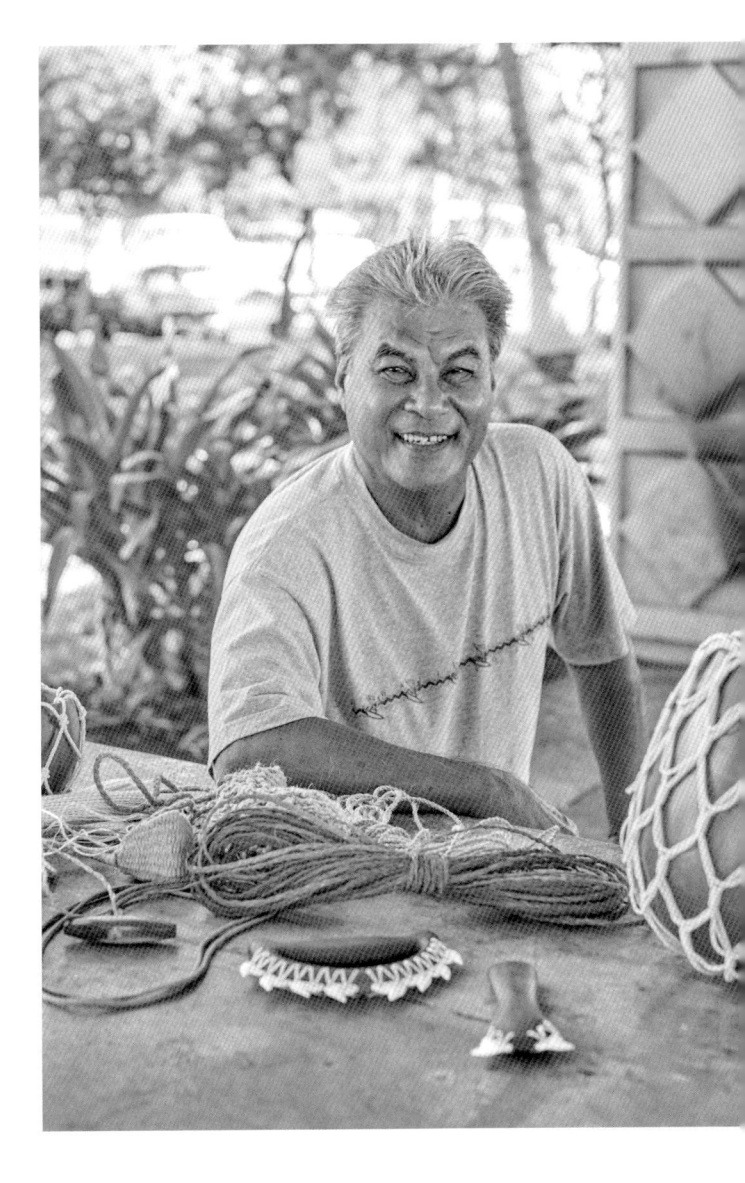

In much the same manner that cordage serves to bind and hold—whether lashing a canoe, netting a gourd, or attaching a weapon—Sonny believes that cordage can symbolically bind our generations. Learning kaula can connect past, present, and future generations in a continuum of cultural pride and cultural esteem.

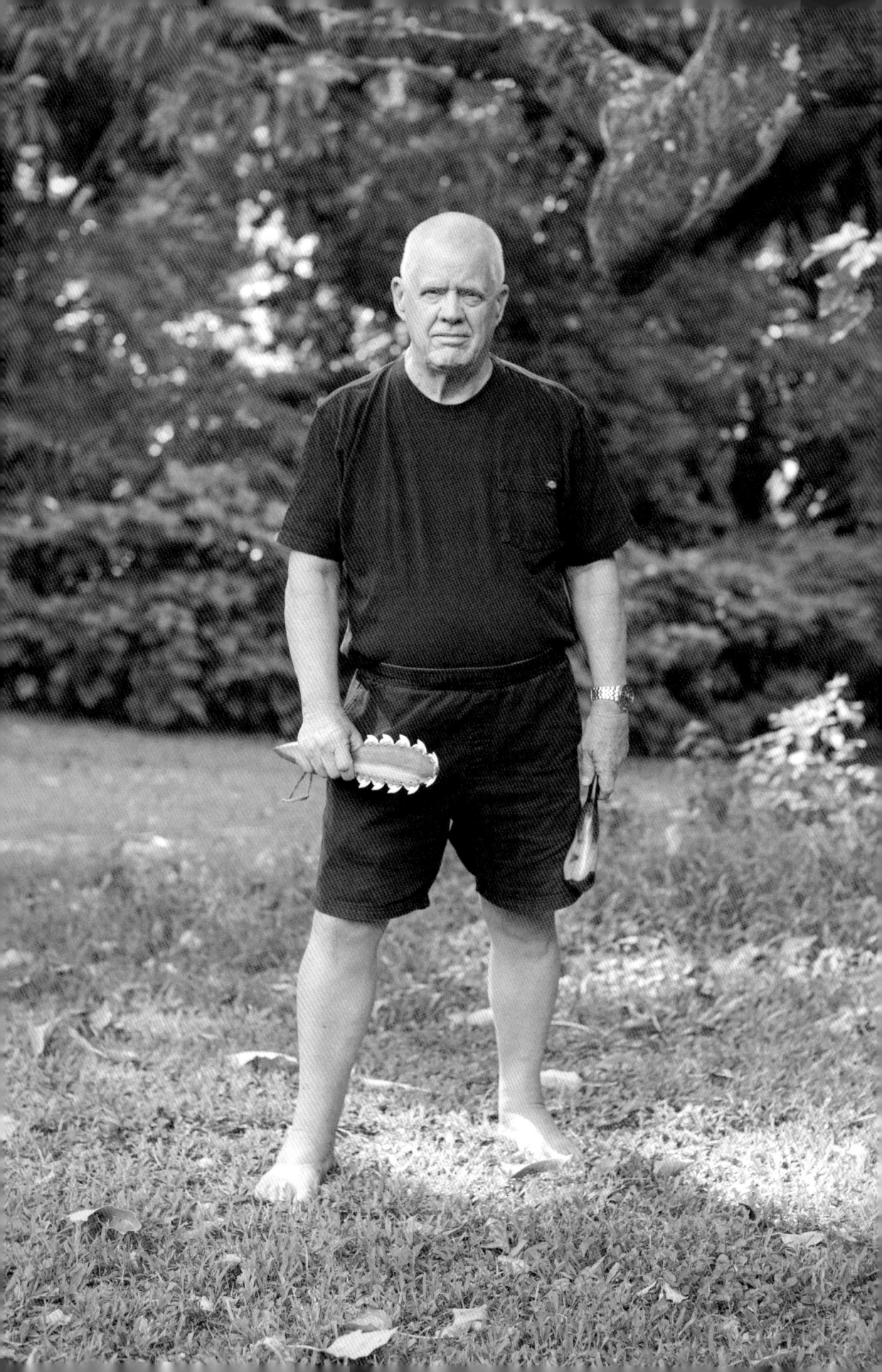

CHAPTER 12

Jerry Walker

LUA

J erry Walker is an accomplished man who heeded the kāhea (call) to teach lua, the Hawaiian art of fighting. Lua is a deadly fighting system that emphasizes bone breaking through hand-to-hand combat and weaponry. In being an ʻōlohe lua, Jerry acknowledges that lua is more than a martial art, it is "a way of life." This "way of life" requires living in harmony with the dual energy sources embodied by two primary gods, Kū and Hina: "Hawaiians combined the art of fighting with ideas of duality and polarity and so embodied lua in two of their primary gods, Kū and Hina, ruling the universe in perpetual balance. Kū: male. Hina: female. Kū: the east and the rising sun. Hina: the west, the setting sun, and the moon. Kū: to stand erect. Hina: to recline, or lie down from being upright. Kū: vertical line, north-south longitude marker. Hina: horizontal line, east-west latitude marker. Kū: right. Hina: left. Their realms embrace the earth, the heavens, and all human generations, past, present, and yet to come" (Paglinawan et al. 2006, 9).

Heeding the Kāhea

Living in harmony with dual energy sources seems an insurmountable task. However, for Jerry, it makes impeccable sense in a fighting art that relies on both male and female energy and force and counterforce. He views lua as a sacred fighting art system meant to protect self, family, chiefs, and gods, and he takes his kuleana of the preservation and perpetuation of lua seriously.

Based on his efforts to preserve this Hawaiian tradition, he was recognized by the Office of Hawaiian Affairs in 2018 with the Nā Mamo Makamae o Ka Poʻe Hawaiʻi (Living Treasures of the Hawaiian People) award. This award recognizes living master practitioners and knowledge keepers in the Native Hawaiian community.

Jerry's stature as an ʻōlohe lua has been influenced by specific circumstances and events in his life. These include his family lineage, his education in the health field, his experiences in the military, and his training in martial arts. Like many Kānaka who want to better understand their cultural identity and history, Jerry searched vigorously for genealogical documentation of his lineage. His genealogy is like that of many persons in Hawaiʻi in its mixture of Kānaka and non-Kānaka bloodlines, but it differs from most people in its chiefly origins.

Jerry's father came to Hawaiʻi from Missouri in the 1940s and married his mother, who traces her ancestry to the royal family of Kamehameha I through Kamaeokalani-wahine. Along with Charles Ahlo, and with oversight from prominent historian Rubellite Kawena Johnson, Jerry wrote the book *Kamehameha's Children Today* (2000). This book documents and chronicles the lineage of Kamehameha I and his wives, who had children who survived into the first and second generations. The book notes that "of the several wives with whom Kamehameha lived, eighteen had surviving children, numbering about thirty, in the first generation" (Ahlo, Walker, and Johnson 2000, 2). The practice of plurality in mating, that is, "for a man to have several wives or for a woman to have multiple husbands," was permissible in premissionary times (Handy and Pukui 1972, 56). For Jerry, this knowledge of his lineage prompted a deeper regard for and desire to perpetuate culture.

Jerry's journey included his education and work in the health field. He earned both a master's and doctorate in public health from the University of Hawaiʻi at Mānoa and worked in population and community health for many years. For example, he worked as deputy director of health for the state of Hawaiʻi; as an administrator for hospitals, including Maluhia and Leahi; and as a deputy director for the Office of Hawaiian Affairs. He also spent twenty-nine years in military service with the US Army, the US Army Reserve, the US Army National Guard, and the US Special Forces as a weapons leader (Danzan Ryu Ohana n.d.).

Throughout his life, Jerry has been an avid student and expert in various martial arts, including judo, aikido, and karate, earning a black belt in kempo karate. His interest in lua began in the mid-1960s, but it took almost a decade before he began to train under one of the few remaining masters of lua. In 1974, Jerry met with ʻŌlohe lua Charles William Luʻukia Kaho Kemoku Kenn in Mōʻiliʻili, Oʻahu. ʻŌlohe Kenn's genealogy of lua is traced to the Kalākaua school and upward to Kamehameha I and Ka ʻAi Kanahā (Paglinawan et al. 2006, ix). ʻŌlohe Kenn also studied with sensei Seishiro "Henry" Okazaki, who incorporated lua into the Danzan-Ryu style of jujitsu. From 1974 to 1978, Jerry trained under ʻŌlohe Kenn with four other Kānaka kāne (Hawaiian men). Early in their training, ʻŌlohe Kenn defined "lua" for them. He explained that "ʻōlohe' had once meant ʻhairless,' from the custom of warriors plucking their hair and greasing themselves so as not to afford the enemy a handhold. The word later also came to mean an expert in any art and a teacher" (Paglinawan et al. 2006, 5).

Training included lectures on cultural topics, field trips to learn about cultural materials such as wild herbs, and training in lua techniques. The discipline and rigor of training earned them the elite status of ʻōlohe lua. At that time, they were given the kāhea from Kenn "to teach, in keeping with the way they had learned, which was the way he had learned, which was the way his teachers had learned" (Paglinawan et al. 2006, 5). When ʻŌlohe Kenn died in 1988, the kāhea to train others became more compelling. This call is reflected in the ʻōlelo noʻeau below, which is the call to prepare for war or prepare for the project at hand.

E HUME I KA MALO, E HOʻOKALA I KA IHE.

Gird the loincloth, sharpen the spear.

(PUKUI 1983, 37)

For Jerry, educational resources include Hawaiian proverbs, and he has identified nearly one hundred proverbs on warriors and warfare from the collection in *ʻŌlelo Noʻeau: Hawaiian Proverbs & Poetical Sayings* (Pukui 1983). Education and training are the ways to perpetuate and preserve lua.

Historical Accounts of the Warrior Way of Life

Feeling an urgency to perpetuate a unique fighting art that was relatively unknown, four of the five ʻōlohe lua (one moved to the US continent) started the training of haumāna in 1993. The imperative to increase the number of people committed to lua is reflected in an ʻōlelo noʻeau that describes the natural color of the pili (grass) being covered by an army of warriors ready for war.

KE ʻULA MAI LA KA PILI.

The pili grass turns red.

(PUKUI 1983, 192)

Training was based on rich historical and cultural information. There are several historical records of lua and warfare in old Hawaiʻi (Cordy 2000; Desha 2000; Kamakau 1964; Malo 1951; Paglinawan et al. 2006), but the highlights below are primarily drawn from the perspective of the ʻōlohe lua who trained under ʻŌlohe Kenn and wrote the book *Lua, Art of the Hawaiian Warrior* (2006)—Richard Kekumuikawaiokeola Paglinawan, Mitchell Eli, Moses Elwood Kalauokalani, and Jerry Walker.

Lua masters existed two centuries before Kamehameha I as small, expert forces of warriors (Paglinawan et al. 2006). In the royal court, the arts of combat were taught and practiced, including spear throwing, pole vaulting, rough-and-tumble wrestling, and boxing (Malo 1951). By the time of Kamehameha I's reign from 1782 to 1819, lua masters had become more proficient, and the art had evolved. In times of war, the lua masters became the battle leaders, supported by the general populace, including farmers and fishermen. Jerry states that approximately "90 percent of the army were regular citizens, and 10 percent were aliʻi." In times of peace, the whole adult male population was a reserve army, each individual of which kept his weapons in readiness in his house: "Training in group fighting was given by the staging of sham battles on those fairly frequent occasions when the people from all the surrounding districts were gathered for some festivity" (Handy et al. 1965, 233).

Jerry suggests that one reason for the dominance of men in warfare is related to the Hawaiian reality of protecting women who bear children and extend lineage. However, he states that royal women were taught self-defense to protect themselves, and that some women did accompany men in the battlefield. For example, during Kamehameha I's battle at Nuʻuanu, Oʻahu, in 1795 there were aliʻi wāhine (women chiefs) who were on the expedition and engaged in warfare by firing muskets with which they were well skilled (Desha 2000).

Like other cultural traditions, lua was founded on spiritual beliefs and practices. Warfare in general, and lua in particular, had rules and formalities, including prayers, invocations, and ceremonial preparations (Handy et al. 1965). Thus, lua masters were not only proficient in physical skills but also knew the spiritual foundation of their culture: "Kuʻi-a-lua is the principal deity of lua, who takes the form of a poʻo lua (double-headed) or puʻupuʻu lima (double-fisted) god. Two other lua deities are Kuʻi-a-holo and Kū-waha-ilo. Women had their own lua Gods, called Popoki, Kihawahine, Ani, Lauhau, Lowahine, and Hua" (Paglinawan et al. 2006, 37). "Kuʻi-a-lua" literally means "the second blow," and is based on the tenet that throwing the first blow is not honorable but defending with the intent to protect is honorable. In defense there is offense, and accepted outcomes would be the maiming or death of the opponent. ʻŌlohe Kenn explains that "he who throws the first blow can call upon Kuʻi-a-Lua for help and assistance but will not receive it. He who throws the second blow to defend himself can call upon Kuʻi-a-lua for help and assistance and receive help" (Paglinawan et al. 2006, 37). For Jerry, with this approach "one has to know both defensive and offensive moves in order to defend and to know what to defend against. It forces one to find a remedy for disagreement, but to be ready to fight as an act of defense." One proverb that reflects this approach is:

E UHAʻI I KA MAKA O KA IHE.

Break off the point of the spear.

(PUKUI 1983, 46)

The spiritual foundation of lua is reinforced by three principles (Paglinawan et al. 2006). The first principle is hoʻomau (perseverance, persistence). It underscores the need for constant practice and repetition such that the art becomes second nature. The second principle is nalu (ocean waves and surf). This emphasizes the benefit of "going with the flow" in order to achieve the balance of duality required in lua. The third principle is hoʻi hou (seeking knowledge by turning to ancestral sources). This requires an openness to receiving such teachings that may lead to greater inspiration and mana.

King Kamehameha I is reputed to have been one of the greatest lua fighters in history. In a demonstration of his skills to British captain George Vancouver, Kamehameha I is said to have "had six spears thrown at him simultaneously and with full force. He caught two, parried three and deflected one" (Kāne 1997, 49). His reputation was most clearly earned, as he relentlessly and strategically unified the Hawaiian Kingdom in 1810 using the lua fighting art, as well as weaponry afforded by Western contact. Despite a transition to Western fighting methods, lua continued to be practiced under Kamehameha I, and he established three schools to further the art. The last words uttered by Kamehameha on May 8, 1819, were:

Ē NAʻI WALE NŌ ʻOUKOU E NĀ ALIʻI,
I KUʻU PONO AʻU I NAʻI AI ʻAʻOLE LOA E PAU.

Endless is the good I have conquered for you.

(DESHA 2000, IV)

Eventually, due to significant cultural changes and transitions, the practice of lua declined.

Revitalizing Lua for the Modern Warrior

Four ʻōlohe lua who trained under ʻŌlohe Charles Kenn established the school Pā Kuʻi-a-Lua in 1993 as their way to honor the kāhea to bring back, revitalize, and perpetuate this ancient fighting art. Like other schools that evolve over time, by the late 1990s, the Pā split into two schools, Pā Kuʻi-a-Lua and Pā Kuʻi-a-Holo. Jerry became a part of Pā Kuʻi-a-Holo with Mitchell Eli. Jerry and Mitchell believed that the classroom, as in old Hawaiʻi, should be in nature—ocean, mountains, forest, and streams. Haumāna and teachers would gather in sites with deeply rooted historical significance, such as Nuʻuanu, Oʻahu, the famous battlefield where Kamehameha I conquered the island of Oʻahu. Jerry states that Kamehameha I and his warriors advanced to "wound Kalanikūpule, the King of Oʻahu and kill Kaʻiana, a renowned warrior chief." They forced the Oʻahu army to the cliffs at Nuʻuanu Pali, where they either jumped or were pushed over the edge.

Training included a forty-eight-hour course over a three-week period. Subsequent and advanced training occurred at other sites. With the Nuʻuanu valley and mountains serving as the classroom, the chanting of haumāna would piercingly reverberate throughout the natural land site. With ferocious concentration, haumāna would chant and practice combat moves by centering the power of their bodies with strikes, punches, and kicks. Jerry tells us that lua warriors will chant the line "Ina kaua e Kuʻi-a-lua" (Fight with me, Kuʻi-a-lua) in their incantation to the deity Kuʻi-a-lua to help them in battle. The spiritual tenet is that the warrior who strikes the second blow will be heard and helped. Haumāna were reminded that the kuʻi ʻakahi (first blow) is the mark of a false warrior (Paglinawan et al. 2006). Chants and prayers helped the warrior prepare inwardly, and they inspired confidence with the belief of Godly support and protection. It is noteworthy that schools today do not require students to worship the lua gods but do request that students respect this spiritual foundation and learn and acknowledge how it relates to this fighting art (Paglinawan et al. 2006).

Learning lua ʻai (lua techniques) is the critical basis for combat training. "ʻAi" also means "to eat." In context of lua, it refers to consuming the enemy by using techniques to maim and kill. Techniques may vary from school to school, but "the four ʻŌlohe of Pā Kuʻi-a-Lua and Pā Kuʻi-a-Holo have identified 359 ʻai" (Paglinawan et al. 2006, 48). The fingers, fist, elbow, ball of the foot, heel, and knee were the means that the lua warrior would use to execute lua ʻai, with calculated moves that involved hitting with a closed fist, chopping with the side of the hand, poking the eyes, breaking the fingers, and squeezing as in a vice hold. Jerry indicates that the "five senses of touch, sight, hearing, smell, and taste were all important in lua, but in addition, the sixth sense of situational awareness was significant, so that one was in a constant state of alertness to stimuli and signals that could indicate a potential danger."

There are many different traditional weapons used in contemporary lua training, including the pololū (long spear), ihe (short spear), pāhoa (dagger), lāʻau pālau (long club), newa (short club), leiomano, kaʻane, and maʻa. "In Hawaiʻi, spears appear to have been the most popular weapons in war" (Hiroa 1957, 418). One type of spear was six to eight feet in length with a thickness that tapered into rows of barbs, and the second was nine to eighteen feet long that terminated with a point similar to a dagger. The leiomano, with shark's teeth, was shaped almost like an oval hand mirror and used to cut an opponent. It was used only to cut up human bodies, and never for other work (Paglinawan et al. 2006).

Intensive training in a spiritual foundation, hand-to-hand combat, use of weapons, fighting formations, and other subjects, such as nutrition and health, would culminate in tests demonstrating knowledge and skills. A sham battle between two sides, each reaching for victory, was an ultimate test. With the successful completion of the sham battle, graduation with a ceremonial pani would symbolize a connection to the ancestral origins of lua and signal a closure of the forty-eight-hour intensive training.

Jerry estimates that since the beginning of training over twenty-five years ago, there have been at least two thousand students who have undergone the initial training. We might expect this number to be larger, since there are other schools of lua. In 2007, Jerry, along with others, started another group called Pā Ka'ai Kanaha Elua, with an interest in research as well as refining training and education in lua.

Preserving the Warrior Way for the Future

Jerry is clear that education and training are important to the preservation of lua for future generations. In the last two decades, the branching of the schools with genealogical links to ʻŌlohe Kenn suggests an increase in varying perspectives and practices. Evolution and diversity are indicative of adaptation to contemporary times, without sacrificing authenticity. Combined with the growth of other lua schools with different lineages, there is evidence for sustaining a sacred practice.

With other ʻōlohe, Jerry agrees that the fighting art of old Hawaiʻi, with its hand-to-hand focus, will not be the future warfare method of choice given technological advancements, new weaponry, and combat modes. A core part of the practice today is historical and ceremonial. There is clear value in learning this ancestral practice as a means to understand Hawaiian roots and identity. However, lua also has the added value of practicing self-defense and developing pono leadership for future generations.

As a martial art, lua provides ample opportunity for training in a form of self-defense that strengthens body, mind, and spirit. Physical exercises in lua, like any other demanding physical workout, builds bodily strength and increases stamina through consistency and repetition. It requires a mindfulness of approach and a razor-sharp focus on fighting techniques. All this is amplified when the lua participant is connected to the lua deities or to other higher powers. In watching a lua demonstration during the Makahiki, a time

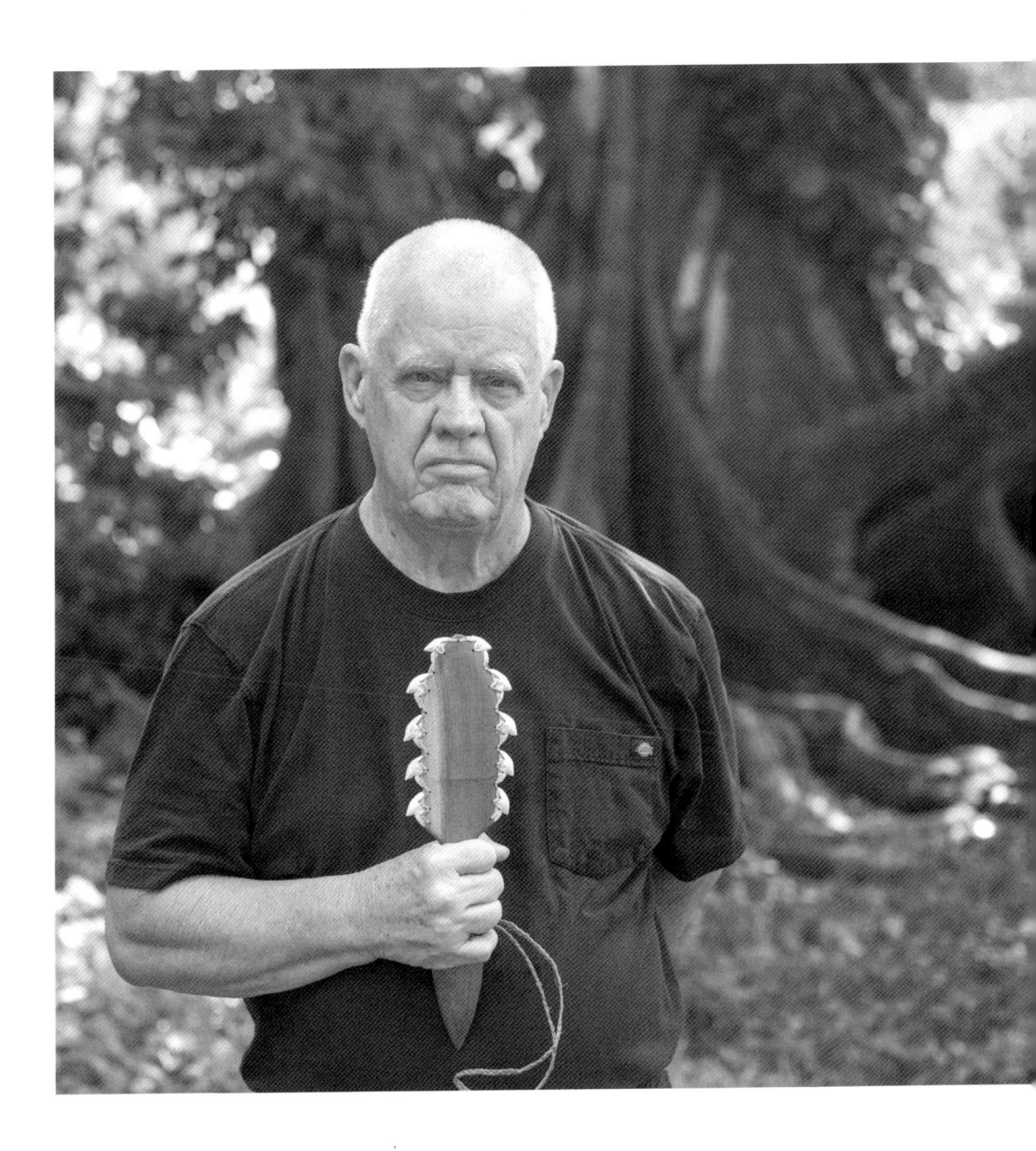

of thanksgiving and ceremonial competition, lua participants mimic the pig grunt of the Kamapua'a (a pig demigod associated with the Hawaiian God Lono) in a deep breathy sound as they execute combat moves. One can imagine the fierceness and physical prowess of warriors from the past: "Ha, he, hu! Ha, he, hu! Ha, he, hu!" There is a "guttural chorus of breathing, each breath inhaled and expelled in an explosive mantra. . . . They lunge forward and back, dodge from side to side, then whirl and pivot in unison, as arms strike aim for an invisible opponent's eyes, then throat" (Sodetani 2003, 1).

While it may not make intuitive sense that someone dedicated to the health field would also be passionate about martial arts, and specifically lua, Jerry reminds us that lua training promotes the development of pono leadership. Anchored in the perspective that lua is a "way of life," pono leadership is about the interdependence of duality and polarity. Recognizing and respecting these opposite forces helps one see both sides and results in a balanced perspective. "Without such a balance comes trouble" (Paglinawan et al. 2006, 10). Fundamental conditions leading to this balance include being rooted in Hawaiian culture, performing the responsibilities of the Hawaiian warrior, and striving to be and acting pono. Lua leaders of today and tomorrow use a spiritual foundation to function in both the Hawaiian community and the broader world.

Lua has relevance for social justice and health equity. By perpetuating its existence as a sacred ancestral practice, there is resistance to historical forces that sought its extinction, and assertion of social justice through its preservation. Jerry's background in health and martial arts is illustrative of the duality expressed by the deities Kū and Hina, and underscores the importance of balance for health and wellness. Health, with its focus on healing, and martial arts, with its focus on combat, appear to be diametrically opposed. But in lua they are reflective of dual elements that are interdependent. A healthy warrior will be a strong warrior, and a strong warrior must know how to heal those who are injured in combat. Jerry clarifies that balance included more than combat medicine and fixing people that are hurt or injured. He says, "What's more important is that you go to the healing side to help balance individuals" so that they can live in appreciation of the Kū and Hina within themselves. For example, he states that warriors who are trained to develop their prowess in battle also compose poetry, dance, surf, and excel in sports and games.

Having honorably answered the kāhea to perpetuate lua through training and education, Jerry now finds that his journey as ʻōlohe brings him to another pivotal juncture. ʻŌlohe are getting older, there is a branching of lua schools, and recent classes may be dwindling in size. Jerry notes that perpetuation will require a kāhea to future generations. This kāhea would emphasize a "way of life" and a fighting approach for elite warriors who are pono and in a balance with dual energy sources. Sharing the following lua declarations, Jerry states that the kāhea continues:

Ua ala a kūʻē!	*They arose and revolted!*
Kūʻē! Kūʻē!	*Revolt Revolt!*
Kamamaka kaua.	*The elite fighting warriors.*

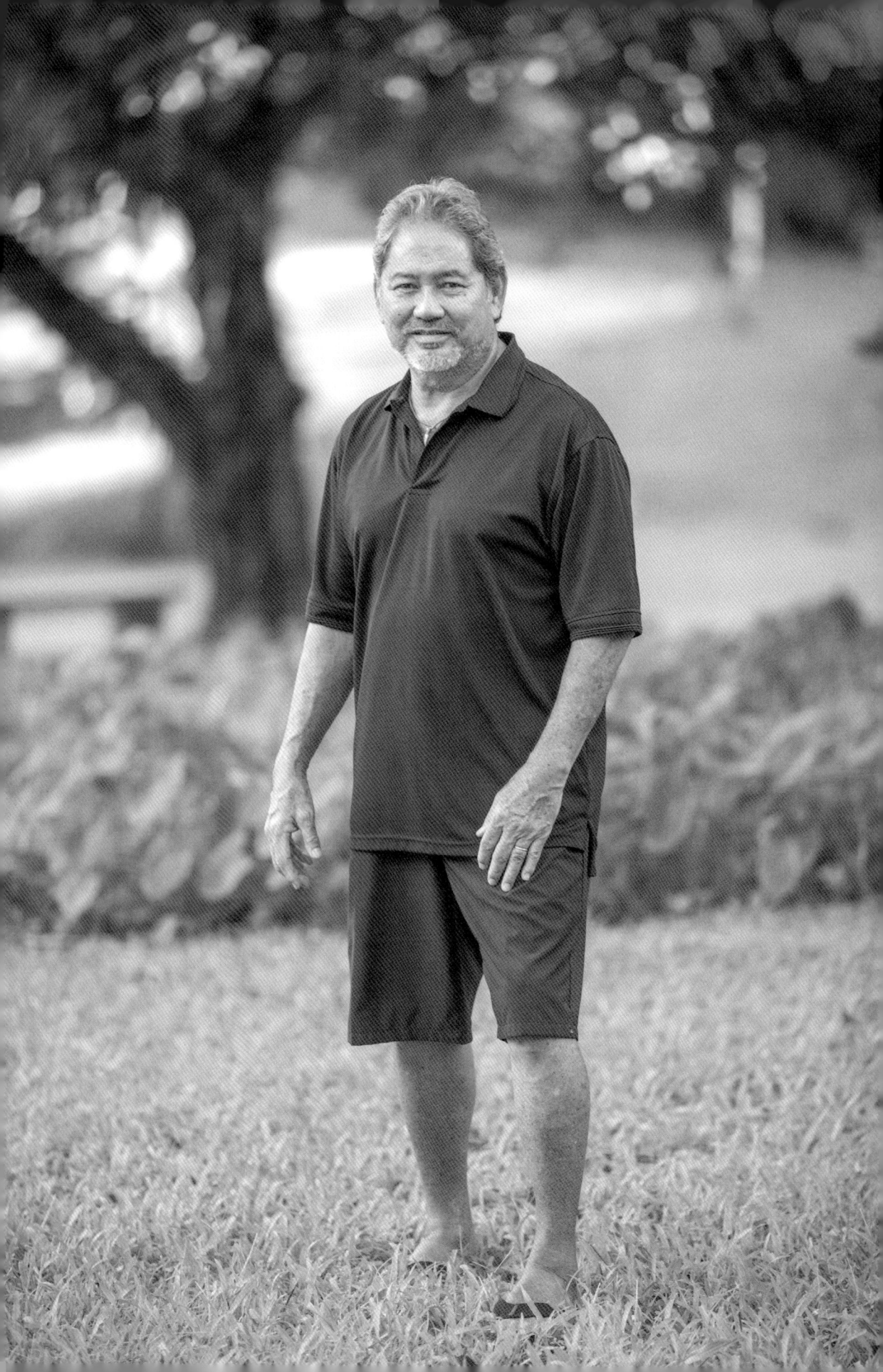

CHAPTER 13

Gordon "'Umi" Kai

NĀ MEA KAUA

Gordon 'Umialiloalahanauokalakaua ('Umi) King Kai descends from 'ohana with roots in Waimea and Waiohinu on the island of Hawai'i. He greets in the traditional style of his kūpuna, with the exchange of hā (breath), ihu (nose) to ihu. This style of greeting is called honi, and requires physical touching in a manner that signifies closeness and intimacy (Handy and Pukui 1972; Kanahele 1986).

'Umi is a man of many skills and talents. He is renowned for researching, designing, and engineering nā mea kaua, or, as 'Umi defines, it "things of war and weaponry." These include long and short spears, daggers, war clubs, adzes, shark-tooth weapons, tripping weapons, slings, and other weapons. 'Umi's passion and expertise in Hawaiian culture, however, encompass a much broader calling, to mea Hawai'i, or Hawaiian things. 'Umi states, "Mea kaua and all other mea Hawai'i are vital to the existence of the Hawaiian culture."

Cultural Identity Anchored in Relationships

Some people have culminating experiences that spark passion. There is a feeling deep in the na'au that one cannot ignore. The journey began early for 'Umi. Moments of cultural significance, living in and visiting other places, and cultivating connections with people all played a part in 'Umi's journey. He recalls several events in his life that shaped his trajectory.

'Umi's first exposure to nā mea kaua occurred when he was a youth. Visiting the home of an uncle, 'Umi was mesmerized by the weapon that was prominently displayed on a wall in the house, a weapon that everyone knew was never to be touched. The weapon was a leiomano, which in cultural tradition "was only to cut up human bodies, never for other work" (Paglinawan et al. 2006, 58). Not too long after that first encounter with the leiomano, 'Umi's uncle passed away, and the treasured weapon was buried with him. On occasion, the image of the leiomano would find its way into 'Umi's thoughts and inspire him to think about a future in which he could make his own weapons.

'Umi spent a good portion of his senior year in high school living in Alaska. The people in 'Umi's new school and new town were fascinated with and curious about this new visitor, who had come across a vast ocean from the small islands of Hawai'i. "They [students, teachers, family, friends] would ask me so many questions about Hawai'i and Hawaiian things," 'Umi states. The allure of Hawai'i is not a new thing, and in fact dates back centuries. Lili'uokalani (1898) wrote about the surge of curiosity that swept the United Kingdom in the spring of 1887, as she and Queen Kapi'olani traveled to London to attend Her Majesty Queen Victoria's grand jubilee. Princess Ka'iulani also wrote about her travels abroad and the curiosity she met along the way. As they traveled, they all remembered feeling genuine pride in being Kanaka, and they felt honored to represent Hawai'i. In 'Umi's case, a deep yearning for cultural knowledge emerged very strongly when he was away from the islands. "It was then that I decided I wanted to learn more."

'Umi returned from Alaska to complete his senior year at Kaimukī High School, and his passion for mea kaua and mea Hawai'i continued. Growing up in the Kaimukī area, he spent much of his time down at the beach. Walking to and from the beach, as most kids did in those days, 'Umi met and learned from two people who became instrumental in his early acquisition of Hawaiian knowledge. He learned through watching and imitating.

I KA NĀNĀ NO A 'IKE.

By observing, one learns.

(PUKUI 1983, 129)

One of his teachers, Ms. Keawe, worked at Pākī Hale just mauka of Kapi'olani Park, teaching malihini (tourists) to make simple lau hala bracelets and coconut hats. 'Umi spent a significant amount of time with Ms. Keawe as she taught the malihini, and he began to learn through observing and eventually replicating her work. As a young Hawaiian man with a heightened new interest, 'Umi learned quickly and soon found that he was teaching the malihini himself, with Ms. Keawe's guidance.

On those same walks, ʻUmi met a Hawaiian man who became another teacher for him: "Talbert George made trinkets, among other things, out of cordage and shark teeth, also for the malihini." The lasting impression left by the earlier encounter with the leiomano, combined with the months under the tutelage of Ms. Keawe, culminated in ʻUmi feeling ready to make his first weapon. After mustering the courage to ask the Hawaiian man if he could purchase some shark teeth, ʻUmi did just that. "Whatchu' goin' do wit' 'um?" the man asked. "I'm going to make a leiomano," ʻUmi replied. This skilled artisan clearly felt that ʻUmi was ready to perpetuate Hawaiian craft making, and provided him with the valuable shark teeth. ʻUmi says jokingly, "In school, woodshop was my favorite subject, and one I could excel in." ʻUmi taught himself and successfully completed his first of many leiomano in his senior year.

After graduation, ʻUmi became close friends with George Helm, a Hawaiian musician who also became a powerful activist for Hawaiian people. Both men had a shared aloha for Hawaiian culture, as they traveled to Japan with a Polynesian group to sing, dance, and play music. Upon their return to Hawaiʻi, their relationship grew stronger as they attended and boarded together at the Church College of Hawaiʻi in Lāʻie. George introduced ʻUmi to Kahauanu Lake, a well-known and respected Hawaiian singer and songwriter steeped in cultural knowledge and traditions.

The relationship with Kahauanu Lake proved to be a pivotal milestone for ʻUmi, as it deepened his understanding of family in the context of culture. Training by many kūpuna often takes the form of questions in which the learner is not provided with the answers but is instead asked to seek answers, and so it was with ʻUmi and Kahauanu Lake. ʻUmi recalls his first conversation with Kahauanu Lake vividly:

"What is that ring on your finger?" he asked.

"It's a gift from my mother," ʻUmi replied. "It has my name [ʻUmialiloa] on it."

"Is that so?" Kahauanu replied. "What does it mean?"

"I don't know," ʻUmi replied.

"Go ask your mom and come back," he said.

ʻUmi went to see his mom that very night and asked her for the meaning of his name. All she could tell him was that it belonged to his grandfather. When ʻUmi went back to see Kahauanu, he was instructed to find the book titled *Ruling Chiefs of Hawaii* (Kamakau 1961), to read the story of his name, and to return and report his findings. Kahauanu then asked ʻUmi a single question that would lead to the solidifying of their lifelong relationship as 'ohana: "Who's your mom?" 'Umi gave the name of his mom as Rachel "Lahela" King Kai of Waimea, Moku o Keawe.

It was then that Kahauanu revealed to 'Umi their shared mo'okū'au-hau through their mothers. 'Umi then became one of Kahauanu's keiki hānai (fostered or adopted child), and would visit with him at his home every Saturday morning to talk about Hawaiian "stuff." Thus, Kahauanu started 'Umi on a journey of self-discovery, through which 'Umi uncovered family stories, riddles, and feelings of triumph, loss, love, resentment, friendship, and adventure. Ultimately, the journey provided the context for 'Umi to obtain a deeper understanding of himself and fueled his passion for mea Hawai'i. Kahauanu's teachings made pa'a the foundation from which 'Umi's life's work would be reflected.

Over the years, 'Umi learned and studied various aspects of Hawaiian culture from other revered culture keepers, including Makahiwa Lua, Wright Bowman Sr., Dr. Yoshi Sinoto, Patrick Horimoto, George Fujinaga, and 'Ōlohe Richard Paglinawan. Under the leadership of 'Ōlohe Paglinawan, 'Umi learned lua and the lifestyle that accompanied it. Historically, a chief's highest class of warriors were the 'ōlohe lua, who were primarily of the ali'i rank and practiced and taught lua. This select group of individuals lived a strict and rigorous lifestyle designed to cultivate and achieve optimum levels of physical, mental, and spiritual agility. 'Umi attended his first lua class out of pure curiosity and then became a lifelong student, stating, "Lua filled a void I didn't know was there" (Sodetani 2003, 32). Learning lua reinforced and complemented 'Umi's passion for making nā mea kaua: "'Umi Kai has become particularly well-known for the quality and terrifying beauty of his weapons. Kai was an accomplished stone and wood carver even before he began practicing lua. Kai's finely crafted weapons have frequently been sought by art exhibitors and private collectors, but he stresses that they're not decorative. They're made for function, not beauty" (Sodetani 2003, 32). Lua training provided for the natural and intrinsic blending of the Hawaiian fighting art with the making of Hawaiian weapons. In 2002, 'Umi joined the ranks with his kumu, earning the prestigious title of 'ōlohe lua.

History as a Basis for Nā Mea Kaua

When the Polynesian wayfinders settled in Hawai'i, they lived in peace for many generations. With the abundance of rich, fertile land, none needed to envy his or her neighbors (Mitchell 2001), and for fifty-three generations, families governed themselves, during which time no man "was made chief over another" (Kamakau 1964, 3). As the population grew, Hawaiʻi eventually became established as a chief-ruled kingdom, and after this some aliʻi began to look with greed upon their neighbors (Mitchell 2001). Aggressive chiefs made war to control more and more lands. The people of those lands had to defend themselves.

In times of war, the best ʻōlohe lua and ʻōlohe koa (master warrior) would train the makaʻāinana in various aspects of lua, including techniques in bone breaking, spear throwing, wrestling, boxing, and pressure point and nerve center manipulation (Mitchell 2001). In general, women were not trained to fight. However, there were women known as koa wāhine (brave women) or wāhine kaua (battle women) who were taught by the men and fought alongside them.

Traditional war making in Hawaiʻi was an intimate affair that included hand-to-hand combat and a sophisticated system of grappling arts supported by heavy-impact weapons and weapons that slash and pierce (Cook et al. 2005). ʻUmi explained that the idea of a weapon is relative, meaning relative to you and your resources, training, and expertise. He states that "the first weapons for the lua practitioners are his hands, and another weapon is prayers." Some practitioners could pray a person to death. A weapon is relative to what you have in your hand or what is available nearby. He continues, "To Hawaiians, a stone or a stick could be a weapon. Other natural materials could also be combined and fashioned for specific functions such as a newa or leiomano. The farmer's main tool, the ʻōʻō, is a perfect weapon; a pōhaku kuʻi ʻai could also be used as a newa. Our kūpuna lived in a warriorship environment. Aliʻi would wipe out entire ahupuaʻa, sometimes entire moku [district, place, island] to ensure that no one could seek revenge. This tells us that everyone had to fight. From aliʻi to kauwa [servants], all who were able took to battle."

Everyone in Hawaiian society innately understood the importance of knowing how to protect themselves, and this was not taken lightly. Warriors made their weapons of wood, stone, and shark teeth (Hiroa 1957; Mitchell 2001). The following are traditional weapons:

* Pololū are spears made from hardwood, typically nine to eighteen feet long.
* Ihe are shorter spears, typically eight feet long with or without barbed points.

* Pāhoa are daggers made from a single piece of hardwood, pointed at one end. They could be made in a variety of lengths, designs, shapes, and materials.
* Newa are clubs that are typically 3½ to 9 inches long, made from natural root enlargements or a combination of a basaltic lava head, grooved with longitudinal furrows to hold the sennit cord, lashed to the top of a wooden handle.
* Lā'au pālau are longer clubs, usually ten to eighteen inches in length, made of hardwood and polished smooth.
* Ko'i (adzes) are sharp stone blades lashed to wooden shafts and effective club-like weapons frequently used in hand-to-hand fighting.
* Shark-tooth weapons are one of the sharpest cutting tools for Hawaiians made from the serrated edge of shark's teeth, used both ceremonially and in battle. They could contain from one to thirty shark teeth firmly fastened to handles of wood, bone, or fiber.
* Pīkoi (tripping weapons) are used in battle to trip up an enemy as he runs toward or away from you, or to bludgeon an attacker.
* Ma'a are slings made from fiber to hurl ovoid stones at an enemy.
* Nounou (field stones) are used in the art of fighting with stones.

"Weapons could be made personally by each warrior, often under the supervision and guidance of a kahuna whose specialty was weaponry," 'Umi states. The primary cutting tool of the craftsman was the ko'i or stone adze. The ko'i was used to fell trees and fashion them into spears and other weapons. Pōhaku 'ānai (stone polishers) of varying degrees of coarseness were used to smooth and polish the wood, starting with coral limestone, then the skin of sharks and rays, and finally fine-grained basalt. Once the weapon was complete, the craftsman would rub kukui (candlenut tree) oil on the surface to protect it. The time and effort put into creating weapons was so great that the weapons themselves became highly revered, valued, and respected. Decorated warriors often gave names to their favorite weapons and believed they held great mana (Mitchell 2001).

Cook et al. stated, "The release of violence and the spiritual malaise that accompanied war was a psychospiritual matter the Hawaiians addressed in pre- and post-battle rituals . . . culminating with the ritual rebirth" (2005, 121). Traditionally, strict and demanding social and spiritual obligations counterbalanced war making. Warrior societies recognized the physical, emotional, and spiritual effects of violence, and thus implemented healing traditions and cleansing rituals into their human and warrior development practices. The

Hawaiian warrior could be true to his warrior self only if he balanced the making of war with the generating of life (Cook et al. 2005).

Moʻolelo tell of chiefs who ruled with great wisdom and foresight, providing periods of peace and regeneration so their people and the land could rejuvenate (Mitchell 2001). For example, war and work were stopped during Makahiki, the multimonth period of the year between harvest and planting. This period begins on the observed rising of the Makaliʻi over the eastern horizon at sunset. The first phase of Makahiki was a time of spiritual cleansing and offering, followed by a second phase of feasting, hula, and competitive games, showing skills in strength, coordination, and flexibility (Feher, Joesting, and Bushnell 1969).

Translating the Value of Nā Mea Kaua for Today

While weapons and the making of weapons were highly valued in the past, ʻUmi states that mea kaua "often receive negative attention" today due in large part to the limited understanding of their historical role and significance. Mea kaua were not only used to cause harm but also to defend against leiomano. ʻUmi states, "I think it's essential for Native Hawaiians and all people to understand that mea kaua were a basic part of the lifestyle in the past. Perhaps more importantly, the making of mea kaua and mea Hawaiʻi were vital to the existence of the Hawaiian culture and identity."

Understanding the function and necessary components of each mea kaua before making it is a crucial part of the process. Function dictates the material and design. ʻUmi explains,

> Take the leiomano, for example. You have to understand the type of woods that are necessary. You have to understand the type of shark's teeth needed . . . why certain teeth were used, and the protocol that came with gathering materials. Last but not least, you have to understand how to make it functional. All of these elements constitute the making of mea kaua. When we create, whether it'd be a weapon, or a kapa beater [tool to make cloth], a papa kuʻi ʻai, or a pōhaku kuʻi ʻai, the process from contemplation to completion is a journey of self-discovery. It is one that builds self-worth and self-pride. At the end of the journey, a great deal of self-respect and respect for the implement are acquired. Self-respect leads to the respect of others, which in the end, benefits all. It is not the implement itself, as much as it is about the journey and the spiritual, mental, and physical growth that is gained from this journey.

Hawaiians, especially the warriors, understood the importance of the balance between Kū and Hina. Kū, meaning "to stand, upright, erect," presides over the male akua, including their properties. Hina, meaning, "to fall, topple, or lean over," embodies all the female akua and represents the power of growth and (re)production. Not only is Kū defined with and in opposition to Hina, but the absence of either would cause the whole society to suffer: "Kū, the masculine, is always accompanied by Hina, the feminine, and together symbolize the balance embodied in well-being" (Pukui et al. 1979, 128–147). 'Umi explains, "Balance does not always mean fifty-fifty. It very much depends on the audience and the circumstance, whether you'd employ more Kū or more Hina. Once that was understood and mastered, it was easier to interact with people and to navigate everyday situations. You have to understand that you have both. You also have to recognize when it's appropriate to lean on one and not the other. If you didn't have proper balance, it could be very detrimental."

'Umi developed a passion for education and believes that the educational aspects of culture are paramount. He takes advantage of every opportunity to educate people about various aspects of Hawaiian culture. He and his work are well known nationally and internationally through exhibitions, lectures, workshops, and cultural demonstrations. His passion for his work has resulted in numerous prestigious awards that emphasize the perpetuation of Hawaiian culture. In 2019, he was recognized with the Duke's Waikiki Ho'okahiko Award, as well as the Nā Mamo Makamae o Ka Po'e Hawai'i: Living Treasures of the Hawaiian People from the Office of Hawaiian Affairs (OHA). With the OHA award, he is acknowledged as a living master practitioner and knowledge keeper in the areas of haku hana no'eau (artist work), Makahiki, and 'ōlohe lua.

'Umi's broad knowledge, cultural expertise, passion, and willingness to teach provide a unique opportunity for learners of all ages, cultures, and levels of experience to take their own journey of cultural connection and self-discovery.

Connection to Health and Social Justice

One of the many lessons 'Umi learned from lua relates to three main principles: ho'omau, nalu, and ho'i hou (Paglinawan et al. 2006). While all three are important, 'Umi talks about the meaning of ho'omau in everyday life. As a contemporary Native Hawaiian weapons maker with access to modern-day tools, 'Umi acknowledges the value in the process of making traditional weapons.

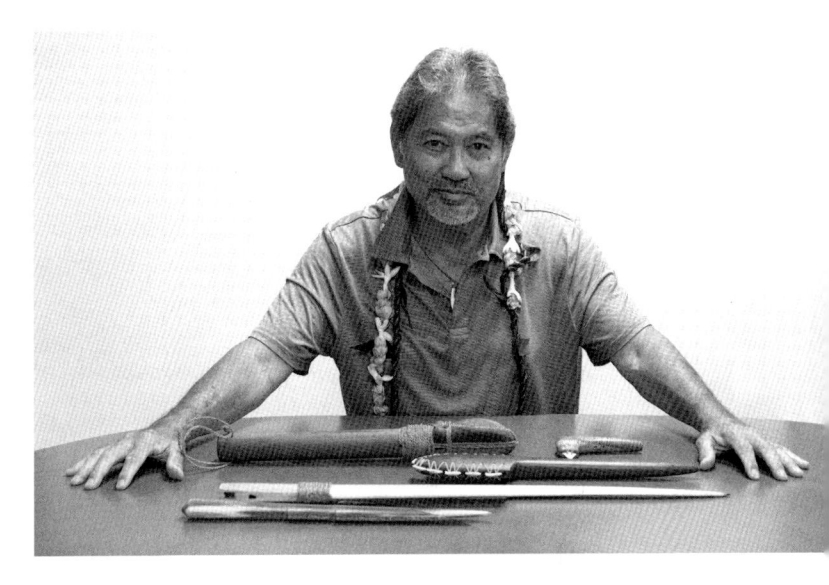

Carving with a koʻi, shaping and sanding with coral and rasps, and chipping and sharpening with stones take time and require effort and patience. But using traditional methods also teaches perseverance and persistence, which then provides a deeper understanding and appreciation of the culture.

Perseverance is not a new concept for Native Hawaiians. Despite the copious historical hardships experienced over the last two centuries, Native Hawaiians maintain their desire and right to thrive. The cultural resurgence that began in the 1970s has gained momentum and continues to connect Native Hawaiians today to cultural traditions that were criticized, condemned, and driven from common practice following Western contact.

Traditional Hawaiian weapon making today is an act of perseverance in perpetuating culture, cultivating pride, and building self-worth. ʻUmi believes that "the creative journey increases self-awareness and cultural resiliency" and a capacity to extend respect to others. He further reminds us that the relationship of self-worth and culture is not new. Kamehameha I, a cultural icon and indisputably the greatest Hawaiian warrior, on his deathbed told his son to e hoʻokanaka (be a person of worth). The last words uttered by a great chief still hold resolute implications for Native Hawaiians today. Living in a constantly changing and unpredictable world, one way to strengthen and build self-worth is to connect to, engage with, and perpetuate cultural practices. The multilayered knowledge found throughout the culture acts as a conduit for Native Hawaiians to return to a source of cultural pride and wellness (Duponte et al. 2010). Helping people to know their worth through cultural connections is gaining momentum. Perhaps the key to the achievement of social justice and better health outcomes for Native Hawaiians lie within the nuances and covert lessons embedded in the Hawaiian culture.

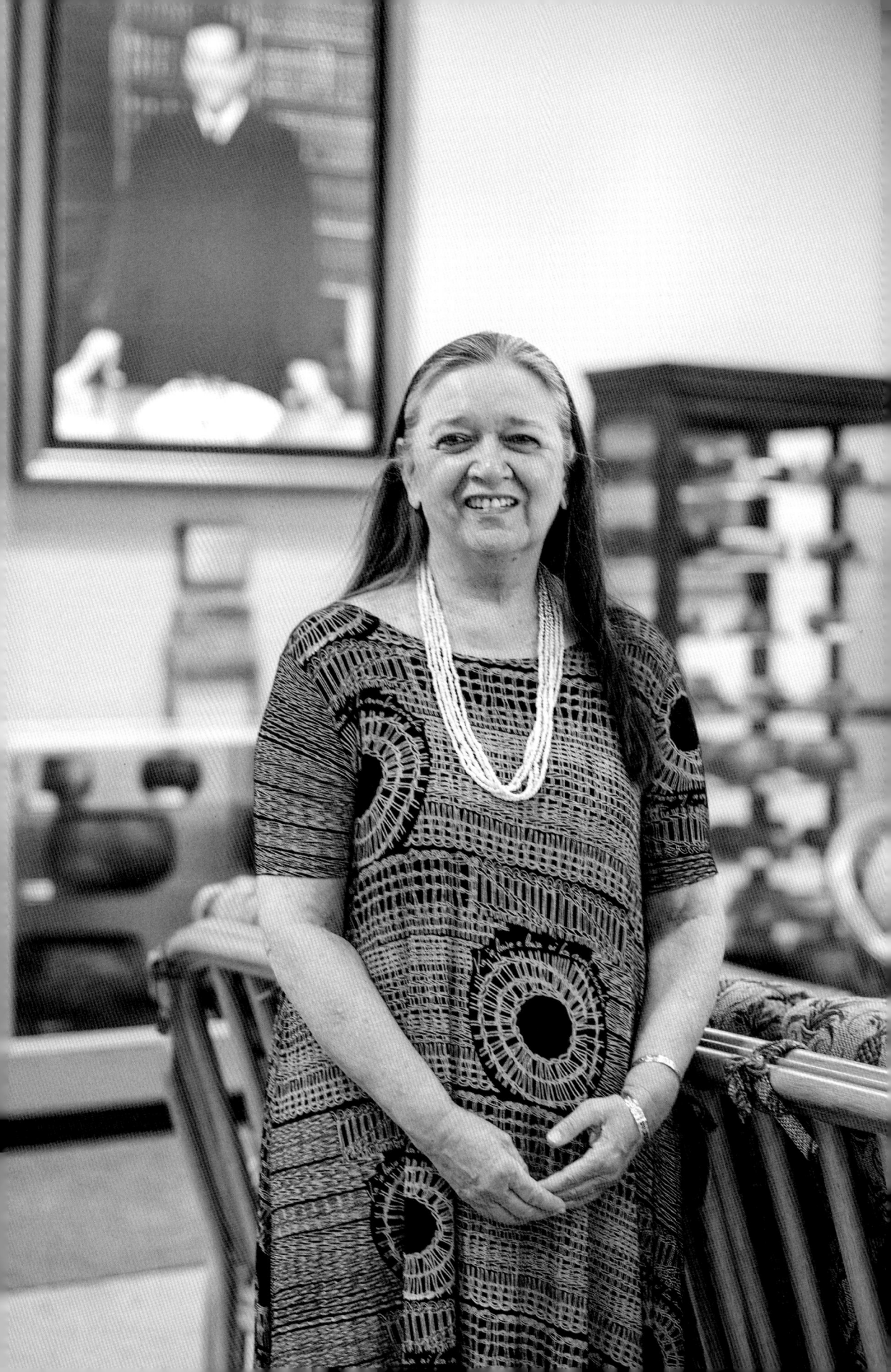

CHAPTER 14

Melody Kapilialoha MacKenzie

NATIVE HAWAIIAN LAW

Melody Kapilialoha MacKenzie understands the distinction and honor of carrying a family name. Her Hawaiian name, Kapilialoha, means "close love" and was given to her by her paternal grandmother, Irene Maluleiliokalani Boyd MacKenzie. As a young child, Melody would ask about the source of her name, but her grandmother would never directly explain it. Rather, over the course of years, through the dropping of hints and ideas, Melody came to understand her name's significance.

Beginning with a Name

Kapili is one of the names of Princess Miriam Likelike and is indelibly linked to the Kalākaua dynasty. As sister to noted siblings King Kalākaua and Queen Liliʻuokalani, Princess Likelike married Archibald S. Cleghorn and had one child, Princess Kaʻiulani. In old Hawaiʻi, it was permissible to engage in "plural mating" (Handy and Pukui 1972, 56), and Archibald Cleghorn previously had a relationship with Elizabeth Lapeka Pauahi Kahalaikulani Grimes, with whom he had three children. One of these children was Melody's grandmother's mother, Helen Cleghorn Boyd.

The distinction of naming and genealogy is further reinforced for Melody, as she knows that a paternal uncle and a maternal aunt also carry the name. In Hawaiian culture, there is great cultural significance in the naming of an individual, as names contextualized and perpetuated kinship networks, expressed love, afforded protection, and provided guidance. In Melody's case, the nomenclature for ancestors establishes permanency of family lineage. It is believed that "the names given to link a child with his or her forebears were of the greatest importance in families of rank. It was and is still customary to give names of forebears, near or distant, for the sake both of identification and commemoration" (Handy and Pukui 1972, 101). Melody also suggests that her name means "loyal" and connotes her kuleana to her family, friends, and community. The gift of the name Kapilialoha set a life course trajectory for Melody that reflects places, relationships, and the duty to seek social justice for Native Hawaiians.

Shaping of Life Direction

Melody's father's family has roots on Maui, and her mom's family has roots on Hawaiʻi Island. But Melody states that the Kailua ahupuaʻa on Oʻahu is considered home. Her parents and two siblings lived with her grandmother, who "had a little bit of land" in Kailua. Knowing the significance and sacredness of names, Melody keeps her grandmother close by wearing a Hawaiian bracelet embossed with her name, Maluleiliokalani.

Melody's grandmother was influential in the sharing of family history that ultimately forged a lineal and personal obligation to helping others. Her stories about the service of Melody's great-grandfather, Colonel James Harbottle Boyd, to King Kalākaua and Queen Liliʻuokalani affirmed the family's historical and cultural links to the Hawaiian community. In addition, the marriage of James Harbottle Boyd to Helen Cleghorn solidified the family lineage to the Kalākaua dynasty. Melody talks about the family story behind the composition of the song "Aloha ʻOe" by Queen Liliʻuokalani. One version of the song's composition states that on a trip to the Boyd estate in Maunawili on the windward side of Oʻahu in the late 1870s, Liliʻuokalani observed a farewell embrace given by James Harbottle Boyd to a young woman. "This tender farewell set Liliʻuokalani thinking, and she began humming to herself on the homeward trip" over the Koʻolau mountains to Honolulu (Gillett 1999, 38). She was inspired to create this song of aloha. It is "probably the best known of all Hawaiian songs" (38):

HUI:	CHORUS:
Aloha ʻoe, aloha ʻoe	*Farewell to you, farewell to you*
E ke onaona noho i ka lipo,	*Fragrant one dwelling in the dark forest,*
A fond embrace, a hoʻi aʻe au,	*A fond embrace then I must leave,*
Until we meet again.	*Until we meet again.*

(37)

The idyllic nature in the creation of this song contrasts with the tumultuous change that was to come with the increased foreign influence in Hawai'i in the late 1880s and the overthrow of the Hawaiian monarchy in 1893. From these stories, Melody states, "we were raised with the idea that we had a familial commitment, a responsibility to work for our community."

Interestingly, the core commitment to the community was expressed in different pathways for the three MacKenzie children in their adult years. Melody's older sister, who has lived away from Hawai'i for much of her life, on the US continent and in South Korea, worked in human resources in the military and is dedicated to the Bahá'í faith. When she returned to Hawai'i, she helped organize a group of Hawaiian language speakers to translate some of the Bahá'í prayers into the Hawaiian language. Melody's younger brother has also lived away from Hawai'i, as he went into the navy after attending the Kamehameha Schools. He settled in Massachusetts, where he worked in a care home facility creating recreational and educational programs. As the lead musician in the family, he has shared his love of Hawaiian music with the patients and the broader community. Melody says that this brother has always been a service-oriented person, committed to helping people in their lives.

Melody's commitment to the community was anchored in her interest in the profession of law and was shaped by her education and work experiences. After receiving her undergraduate degree in comparative religion and anthropology in 1970 from a small college in Wisconsin, Melody moved to Colorado. She began to work in a newly established national law firm, the Native American Rights Fund. Inspired by the work of this organization around the Native American movement and events such as Wounded Knee, Melody decided that her pathway would include going to law school.

She moved to Washington, DC, to attend the Antioch School of Law with its focus on public advocacy and was able to work for representative Spark Matsunaga for a semester. Auspiciously, on a summer break back in Hawai'i, she worked for the Hawaiian Coalition of Native Claims, which eventually became the Native Hawaiian Legal Corporation (NHLC). From this work, she realized that she would have more opportunities to labor for Native Hawaiian causes in Hawai'i than in Washington, DC. So, she transferred to the newly formed William S. Richardson School of Law at the University of Hawai'i at Mānoa (UHM). She graduated with the first cohort from the Richardson School of Law in 1976, with notaries such as former governor John Waihe'e and Honolulu councilmember Carol Fukunaga.

In one of her earliest experiences as an attorney, Melody worked with colleagues such as John Waiheʻe in legal research and strategy for Native Hawaiians. They defended those arrested for attempting to stop the military bombing of Kahoʻolawe and who were seeking to protect cultural and ancestral lands. Although some of these early efforts were not successful in federal court, they put Melody in a community of Native Hawaiian advocates and positioned much of her future work on aloha ʻāina and Native Hawaiian rights.

The mid-1970s was a pivotal time in Melody's life, with her graduation from law school and her early work experiences in Hawaiian advocacy and social justice. It was also a time for her deepening cultural interest in hula. Melody acknowledges that returning to Hawaiʻi to work at the Hawaiian Coalition of Native Claims was "something she wanted to do," but she was also influenced to remain in Hawaiʻi by a pivotal experience related to hula.

Melody was able to attend Māpuana de Silva's hōʻike (presentation) for her ʻuniki (graduation) as a kumu hula under Auntie Maiki Aiu Lake in the summer of 1975. Melody states, "I got to go to her ʻuniki because we had grown up together, and my mom and her mom were close friends. Not many people got to attend this event." Melody says that their families had a close relationship, with their parents often working together on celebrations for the Kailua community. Melody's father was the leader of a group of men constructing and tending the imu (underground oven) for the pig. Her mother, along with Māpuana's mother, and other friends would make Hawaiian dishes, like squid lūʻau (dish with squid and leaves of the taro plant), lomi salmon (dish made from salted salmon, tomatoes, onions, and green onions), and chicken long rice (dish of chicken and rice or bean vermicelli noodles).

Melody's early training in hula began when she and her sister took hula from Francis Beamer when they were growing up in Kailua. Melody renewed that interest in hula when she returned to Hawaiʻi. She began taking classes with kumu hula Māpuana de Silva when Hālau Mōhala ʻIlima was established in 1976. Training was more than just learning about hula; it also reflected the enduring relationship of these two women, close family connections, and a passion for cultural integrity and preservation. With years of disciplined training and practice, Melody graduated as a kumu hula in 1989 and continues to support Hālau Mōhala ʻIlima in teaching and with cultural protocol at special events. More importantly, she sustains a strong relationship with Kumu Māpuana based on reciprocal respect and commitment to the Hawaiian community.

Code of Conduct of Laws in Old Hawai'i

With a commitment to social justice for all people, and a special kuleana for Native Hawaiians, Melody worked at the NHLC as a staff attorney for a decade and as executive director for several years. While there, she wrote significant parts of and edited the first book on Native Hawaiian rights, the *Native Hawaiian Rights Handbook* (1991). With her work experience, Melody began to develop an understanding of Hawaiian history and culture as it pertained to law. The kapu system existed in ancient Hawai'i as a code of conduct of laws and regulations. This system of rules governed "people not only by external force but even more by spirituality" and was fundamentally "designed to prevent spiritual debasement or defilement" (Handy et al. 1965, 39). The discipline of the kapu system could be rigid and severe, but it created order and organization that affected lifestyle, gender roles, politics, and religion. A violation of certain strict kapu could result in death.

Kānāwai (laws) were those edicts that sustained relationships between the spiritual realm, the environment, and people. They could have harsh or beneficial effects. According to Kamakau (1964), "There were two kinds of kānāwai observed by Hawaiian people from ancient days: the kānāwai akua, or Gods' laws, and the kānāwai kapu ali'i, or sacred chiefly laws" (11). Life could be spared by the ali'i.

Melody relays the mo'olelo of the kānāwai that serves as a precept in Hawaiian law—Kānāwai Māmalahoe, Law of the Splintered Paddle. The Kānāwai Māmalahoe was the edict declared in 1797 by Kamehameha I that determined life and death, ensured basic human rights, and protected the vulnerable. It stipulated, "Let the old men, the old women, and the children sleep [in safety] on the highway" (Kamakau 1964, 15). It originated in Kamehameha I's experience in Puna when he pursued a group of fishermen who had something he wanted. While he was chasing them, his foot was caught in a lava crevice. One of the fishermen "lifted his paddle and struck Kamehameha on the head so hard that the paddle was splintered to pieces" (Williams 1993, 58). The fisherman did not know it was Kamehameha, and did not kill him. Years later, the fisherman who struck Kamehameha with a paddle was brought forward to be punished. Kamehameha, understanding his own role in the incident, forgave him and declared the Kānāwai "to protect the weak from the strong" (86).

Native Hawaiian Law Today

Melody states that the William S. Richardson School of Law has the splintered paddle as a symbol and believes that the moʻolelo behind this kānāwai fits in with the mission of the law school in ensuring basic human rights and the protection of the vulnerable. Her relationship with the namesake of the school is personal, as she worked for Chief Justice Richardson after graduating with her degree in law. As she describes him,

> He was . . . an incredible advocate for those who were underrepresented and for the Hawaiian community. He had a strong belief that our laws should not just follow American-European law, but that we had to look at what our ancestors did and how they treated the ʻāina and the water and all of our natural resources. He would tell us that in old Hawaiʻi, the sovereign held the beaches on behalf of all people so they cannot be privately owned today. Similarly, our laws and the courts hold the same position with regard to water and stipulate that water cannot be privately owned. C. J. Richardson was an amazing and compassionate man who understood his responsibility to Hawaiʻi and all of its people.

As the founding director of Ka Huli Ao Center for Excellence in Native Hawaiian Law at the law school, Melody builds on and expands the principles and actions of Chief Justice Richardson and many other legal experts advocating for Hawaiian law.

Native Hawaiian law is that specific body of law that affects Native Hawaiians. The beginnings of this body of law might be traced to the 1921 Hawaiian Homes Commission Act and the 1959 Admission Act, which acknowledged Native Hawaiians as an Indigenous people with distinct rights (MacKenzie 2015c, xi). But Melody states that many aspects of Native Hawaiian law have their genesis in Hawaiian cultural practices, as well as in events during the Kingdom period. In the last several decades, this body of

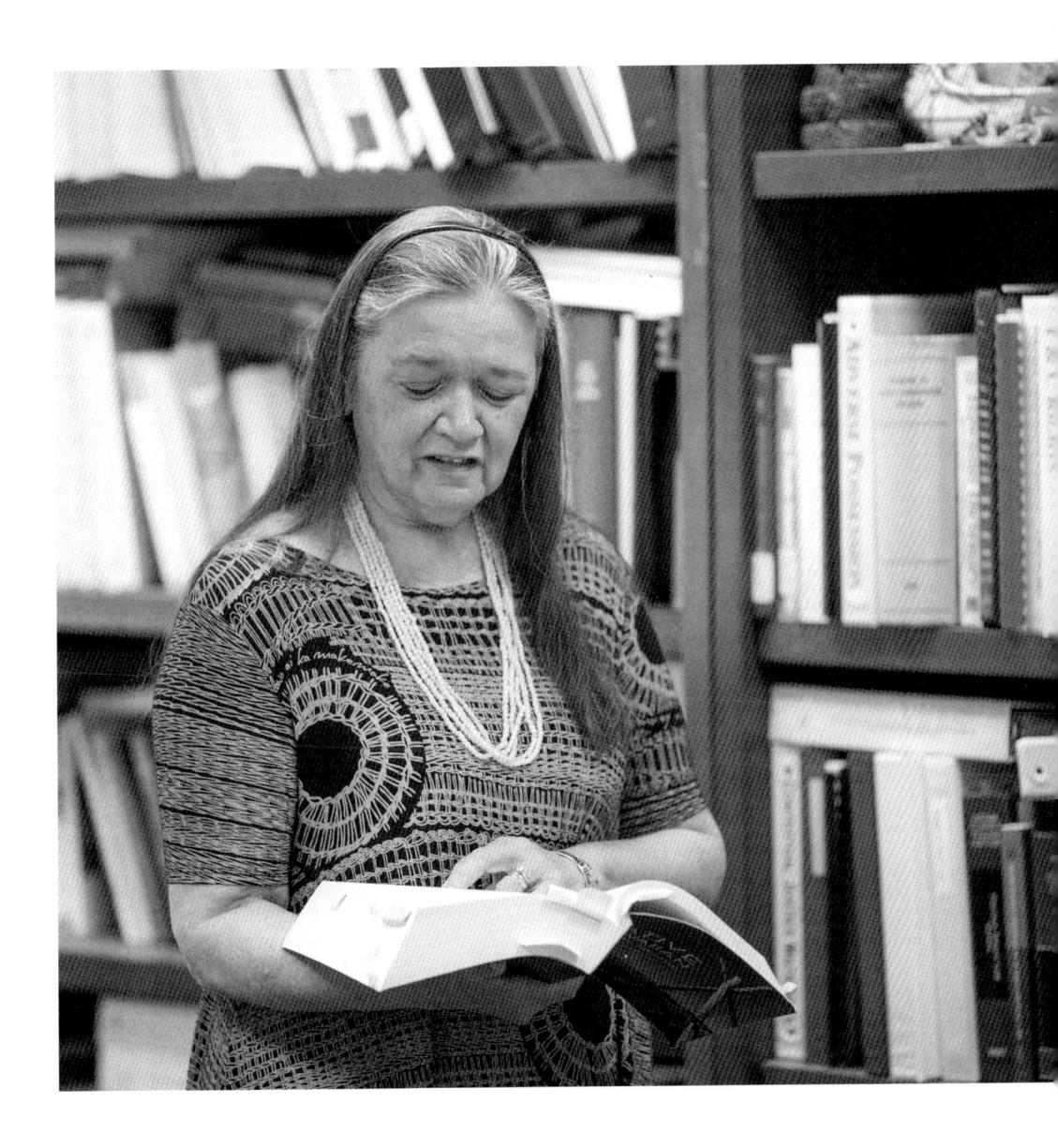

law has evolved in a complex and interrelated manner to recognize the legal and political relationship of the Native Hawaiian people with state and federal governments, and to also explicate general laws pertaining to issues such as access to beaches and shorelines and traditional and customary rights. In 2015, Melody, along with colleagues Susan K. Serrano and D. Kapuaʻala

Sproat, wrote many of the chapters in and edited *Native Hawaiian Law: A Treatise,* a definitive book on critical legal issues for Native Hawaiians. It analyzes events, cases, statutes, regulations, and actions pertaining to the rights of Native Hawaiians. In this treatise, Native Hawaiian Law is organized in the following areas: lands and sovereignty, individual land titles, natural resource rights, traditional and customary rights, and resources for Native Hawaiians (MacKenzie, Serrano, and Sproat 2015).

The following highlights excerpted from this seminal book concern land, specifically the public land trust (MacKenzie 2015b, 76–146; for a comprehensive discourse on the topic, readers are directed to the full chapter). The chapter begins with a statement emphasizing the significance of land to Native Hawaiians: "ʻĀina is a living and vital part of the Native Hawaiian cosmology and is irreplaceable. The natural elements—land, air, water, ocean—are interconnected and interdependent. For Native Hawaiians, land is not a commodity; it is the foundation of their cultural and spiritual identity as Hawaiians" (MacKenzie 2015b, 78). Laws surrounding the ʻāina are of pivotal importance for Native Hawaiians, given the pilina between the land, Kānaka, and the spiritual realm. For Melody, "All are related in a deep and profound way that infuses Hawaiian thought and is expressed in all facets of Hawaiian life" (MacKenzie 2015a, 6). In old Hawaiʻi, there was no private landownership. Through genealogical connections with the spiritual realm, the aliʻi managed the lands that were administered by the kanaka kālaimoku and worked on by the general populace for the benefit of all. In 1848, Kamehameha III set aside Crown lands in the mahele for the income and support of the Crown, and the government lands for the benefit of the people. In 1898, after the illegal overthrow of the Hawaiian monarchy, all of the Crown and government lands, about 1.8 million acres, were "ceded" to the United States. In the 1959 Admission Act, about 1.4 million acres of these Crown and government lands were transferred from the United States to the newly created state of Hawaiʻi.

Notably, the lands granted to the state and the proceeds from the lands were to be held for five trust purposes, including "the betterment of the conditions of native Hawaiians, as defined in the Hawaiian Homes Commission Act" (MacKenzie 2015b, 86). The Hawaiʻi Department of Land and Natural Resources is the state agency primarily charged with the administration of the public land trust. Under this purview, numerous problems have existed over the years, such as the absence of an accurate inventory of trust lands and the failure to account for funds from public lands. The establishment of the Office of Hawaiian Affairs (OHA) following the Constitutional Convention of 1978 was, in part, intended as a correction to problems in that OHA would receive a pro rata portion of the income and proceeds from certain trust lands and would be able to hold title to all real or personal property set aside or conveyed as a trust for the Native Hawaiian community.

There is increasing discussion and some level of progress around trust lands for Native Hawaiians, including some financial benefits to Native Hawaiians and keeping trust lands intact for the foreseeable future. However, significant problems continue to exist. Foremost is the failure to address the underlying claims of Native Hawaiians to government and Crown lands. Central to any discussion are federal and state control and responsibilities in relation to these lands. Examples of other prevailing issues include the US military's use and abuse of trust lands, such as the bombing of the island of Kahoʻolawe, damage from training in Mākua Valley on the Waiʻanae Coast on Oʻahu, and the continuing live-fire training at Pōhakuloa on Hawaiʻi Island. Moreover, questions of how much revenue is generated from trust lands and what portion should go to OHA to benefit the Native Hawaiian community are still contested.

Anchor for Native Hawaiian Law

Ka Huli Ao, the Center for Excellence in Native Hawaiian Law at the William S. Richardson School of Law at UHM, serves as an anchor for Native Hawaiian law in education, scholarship, and service (Ka Huli Ao n.d.). Given Melody's life trajectory and the intersections of law and Native Hawaiian rights, it is easy to understand how she became the founding director of Ka Huli Ao.

The center was established in 2005 through a Native Hawaiian Education Act grant, but as most grants are not intended to be long-term, funding eventually ended. Melody credits the effective work of the Kūaliʻi Council, a campus-wide network representing Native Hawaiians at the UHM, in supporting the sustainability and growth of Ka Huli Ao. The center's educational emphasis is on providing students with ʻike to advance the legal rights of Native Hawaiians and other Pacific and Indigenous Peoples. The center offers the first-ever Native Hawaiian Law Certificate, as well as a rich menu of courses that build on the mandatory course in Native Hawaiian rights.

The center's research and scholarly work emphasize legal learning and incorporate history and culture within a present-day context to advance social justice. The center is deeply invested in service to the community: "Ka Huli Ao facilitates discourse between the legal community, the Native Hawaiian community, and the community at large. Law students and faculty—through workshops, symposia, and meetings—inform and educate, and are educated and informed by, the community about significant Native Hawaiian issues, history, and law" (Ka Huli Ao n.d.). Melody provides examples of trainings for officials and organizational leaders. She states that "training provided to federal agencies, state and county lawmakers, and policy and decision makers as well as congressional staff members are diverse and include many topics. These topics include ceded lands and the public land trust, traditional and customary rights, water and the public trust doctrines, laws relating to kūpuna iwi (ancestral bones), and the state of Hawaiʻi's trust obligations to Native Hawaiians." She also indicates that there are opportunities for monthly discussions and forums on issues important to the Native Hawaiian community. These include "court decisions and laws on Hawaiian immersion education, water rights, the UN Declaration on the Rights of Indigenous Peoples, the protection of cultural and natural resources in Hawaiʻi, the legal challenges and cultural perspectives on Maunakea, and the struggle for Native Hawaiian self-determination."

Melody's imprint on Native Hawaiian law is irrefutable. It starts with genealogical origins and progresses through her experiences with people and places, with attention to the unwavering support of her husband, Lawrence K. Araki, ʻohana, and friends. It culminates in her lifelong commitment to social justice. She is a leader who is humble, gracious, and generally quiet and soft-spoken. However, when the legal debate warrants, she is also a powerful advocate who speaks boldly, and people will listen. She is front and center to building the next generation of lawyers who advocate for social justice for Native Hawaiians. For her lifetime dedication, she has received numerous awards, including the 2006 Hawaiʻi Women Lawyers' Lifetime Achievement Award for her groundbreaking work in Native Hawaiian law, the 2013 University of Hawaiʻi Regents Medal for Excellence in Teaching, the 2020 University of Hawaiʻi Robert W. Clopton Award for Distinguished Community Service in law and social justice, and the 2020 Native Hawaiian Chamber of Commerce ʻŌʻō Award for leadership in education and Native Hawaiian law. Professor D. Kapuaʻala Sproat, a colleague at the law school, eloquently and unequivocally states what many others already know: "When you think about Native Hawaiian law, you think about Melody."

Melody sees the importance of law in helping Native Hawaiians to "chart their own destiny—reviving language and culture, protecting and caring for their lands and natural resources, and seeking ways to restructure the relationship with the United States" (MacKenzie 2015a, 46). Native Hawaiian law, with its tenets rooted in ancestral practices, is a mechanism for social justice.

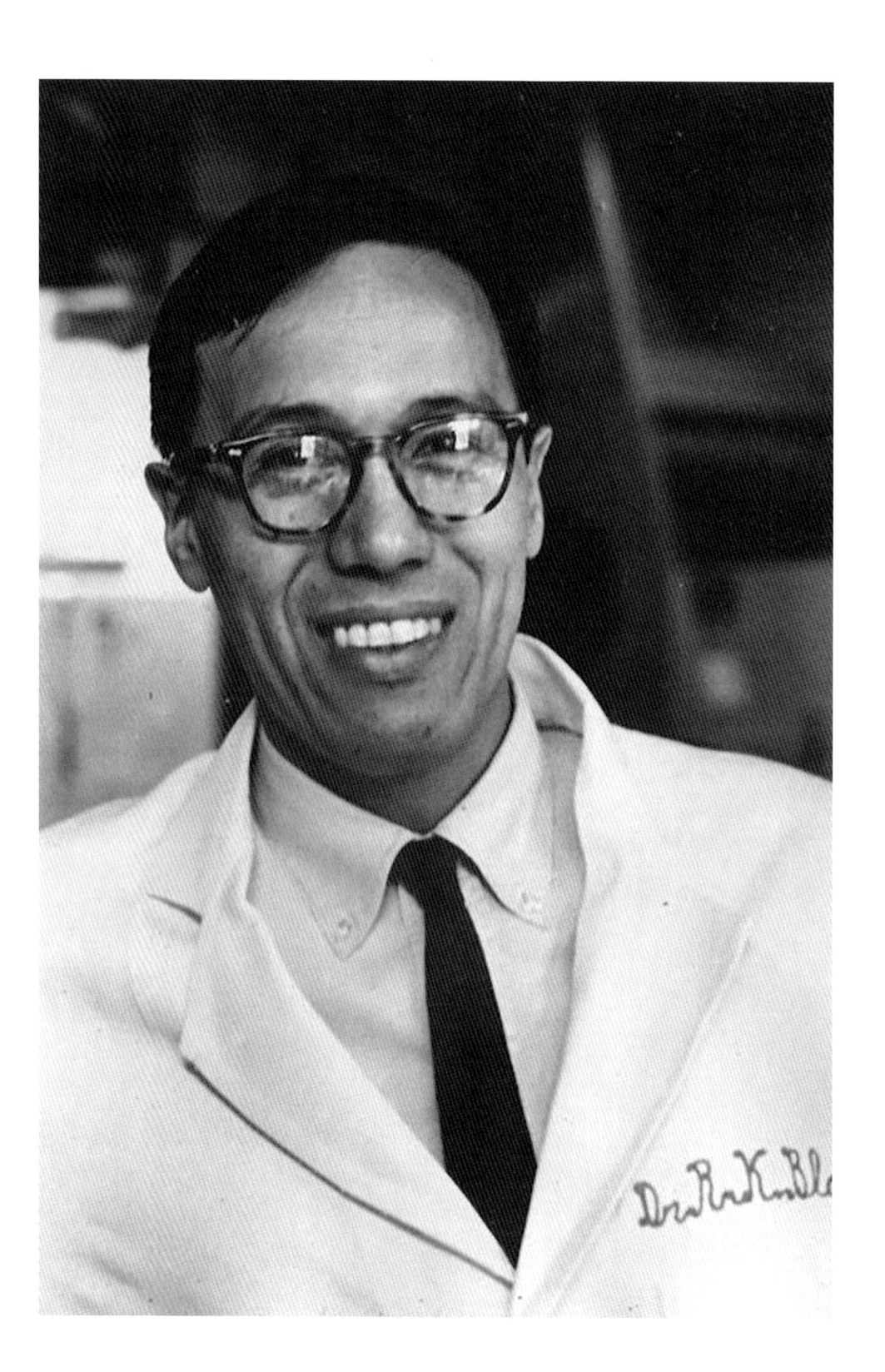

CHAPTER 15

Kekuni Blaisdell

KŪ KA ʻŌHIʻA I KA ʻAʻĀ: ʻŌHIʻA THAT STANDS AMID THE LAVA FIELDS

BY NOREEN MOKUAU, KAMANAʻOPONO CRABBE, AND KEALOHA FOX

With haliʻa aloha (cherished memory) and sincere gratitude, a few of us sat together to share personal reflections about Kekuni Blaisdell, a beloved man who had mentored and nurtured us for many years. The gathering was reminiscent of previous afternoons in Nuʻuanu when Kekuni had welcomed haumāna to his home—a kīpuka where kapa hung on the wall and conversations flowed freely. Memories of these precious times together were still vivid: Kekuni's dark red ink pen to correct our manuscripts, perhaps a camera to capture a moment in time, his reclaiming of the phrase "Kānaka Maoli" to describe the first peoples, his persistent reminder that Hawaiʻi is the "mainland" and, most significantly, his leadership in establishing strong pilina that connect the lāhui and will continue to unite us. The essay that follows is our expression of profound aloha, respect, and appreciation for Kekuni Blaisdell.

Dr. Kekuni Blaisdell's influence is immeasurable. He provided healing to his patients. He generated multifaceted growth in Hawaiian learning throughout the University of Hawaiʻi. He was key in the authorization of the Native Hawaiian Health Care Act through the United States Congress. He always acknowledged that he was standing on the shoulders of others and learning from so many, and he graciously shared his knowledge with whomever he came in contact with.

Kekuni's Kanaka heart knew that relationships are fundamental to our growth as Hawaiians. For decades, he helped to hoʻoulu us from tiny saplings into mature trees. His greatest strengths were in building relationships and nurturing our pilina with each other. To honor this legacy, we strive to remember what Kekuni taught us, reflect his vision for healthy Kānaka, and sound the kāhea to collectively restore our lāhui. Ua hoʻomakua ka lāʻau.

To us, Kekuni is a grandfather figure. For many in the health fields, perhaps hundreds, he is the kupuna we look up to and admire. He was completely invested in helping the lāhui. Kekuni knew that collective action starts simply by coming together; the instant we encircle for "Hawaiʻi Aloha," we are in a position to become agents of change and carry our voices forward. Up until the last "Mau ke aloha, no Hawaiʻi," it was obvious that Kekuni possessed true humanistic waiwai and rich perspectives that amplified Hawaiian values, practices, customs, and beliefs.

The ʻōlelo noʻeau in our title, "Kū ka ʻōhiʻa i ka ʻaʻā," captures Kekuni's essence as a rare individual who, despite challenges, forged a pathway of resilience for others to follow. Similar to the lone ʻōhiʻa tree that sprouts forth in the fresh lava field, he created space for others to take root and follow. Among the core values Kekuni has taught and exemplified throughout his life, the following are those that we aspire to perpetuate now and in the generations to come:

1. **E Hoʻokanaka.** Live as Kānaka Maoli. We must encourage Kānaka Maoli Indigenous distinction and break the cycle of cultural trauma and disintegration of cultural identity.

2. **E Hoʻokahua.** Make Kānaka Maoli strengths and resilience the foundation of our work. Mauli ola is not linear. We must holistically shift the entire deficit paradigm and instead focus on mobilizing our collective strengths toward equity.

3. **E Hoʻokū.** Embrace active use of Hawaiian values and practices. Advocate for the resurgence of our cultural practices, and value spirituality in healing traditions and ola practices. Embed these values in the kahua of your work, articulate them within your practice, and be humble.

4. **E Hoʻokāhuna.** Provide mentoring of Kānaka Maoli. Mentor with deep aloha for one another, as well as for those who came before us. Build up the next generation of Kānaka Maoli experts across disciplines through apprentice-style practices.

5. **E Hoʻōla.** Nurture leadership within the Kānaka community. Rise up and be leaders across organizations in Hawaiʻi. Be inclusive with Kānaka Maoli and non-Hawaiian allies. Lead out with our values and principles to bring us together for the greater good.

6. **E Hoʻoulu.** Build a collective vision that is forward-looking. Create a legacy of Kānaka Maoli solidarity that conveys a greater vision of ola for our people, our homeland, and our ever-expanding waiwai.

Being a Kumu

It is often difficult for a kumu to provide gentle guidance for the students' learning process while simultaneously elevating their practice. Yet Kekuni was able to do this seemingly without effort. Rather quickly, our kumu became our mentor and, later, our friend. He knew us, he knew our ʻohana personally, and he understood our goals.

Kekuni's style captured the essence of being a Kanaka in academia. He cut through the silos that would have kept us divided. He went across disciplines to support Hawaiian haumāna such as ourselves. He facilitated training across many areas of study, even for those who weren't medical students. All Hawaiians at the University of Hawaiʻi knew Dr. Kekuni Blaisdell—he was an integral part of the positive energy around campus and the mana that was building within an institution that had long felt detached from us and our knowledge base.

Being an astute scholar, Kekuni launched a concept that predates the "social determinants of health" model as we know it today. He looked at Native Hawaiian health concurrently through medicine, social work, psychology, nursing, dentistry, and public health disciplines and built his theoretical orientation that we follow today and teach to our own haumāna. Looking back, we cannot think of anyone in our community who constructed that pathway to healthy solutions before he did. Kekuni was a Renaissance man who took his studies from all over the world, from the finest institutions, and returned to Hawaiʻi, as a calling, to bring that intellect forward to help our people. He created a net throughout our community, in which each connection and kūkākūkā made additional knots, expanding the ʻupena and bringing more knowledge and haumāna to strengthen our collective efforts.

Instilling Cultural Esteem and Identity

Instilling cultural esteem was central to Kekuni's style of teaching and mentoring as a kumu. He took special care to cultivate a positive ethnic identity within each of us and stressed it as an important foundation throughout our training. He taught his students to be proud of who we are as Kānaka, in a way that our secondary school teachers did not teach us decades ago—and that certainly was not emphasized during Kekuni's time in the 1940s. Kekuni was a true leader who helped to shift that cultural mindset within many of us. He taught us to be grateful to do this work, and to heal with humility, starting from within. He was intimately aware of the clash of values we were regularly presented with, and he helped us reconcile the loss of Kānaka Maoli identity and self-esteem as health practitioners. He was one of only a few leaders who facilitated that reconciliation for us, perhaps even more than our parents were able to at that time, given their generational disconnect to Hawaiian culture. Some of us didn't have fathers who could speak about hoʻoponopono, or cultural loss, or the importance of Hawaiian spirituality. We saw Kekuni as a role model to guide our parallel process while becoming healthy adults and community leaders.

Kekuni's particular technique of instilling cultural esteem and identity did not allow us to look down on ourselves or see ourselves as "less than." This shade of internal development may not be fully discernable to the current generation of young Kānaka, but for us, it was a genuine struggle to walk in both worlds. Some of us were just trying to survive in a Western world of English, math, and science courses. But with Kekuni, we not only completed those subjects with mastery but also were able to weave in much more while he took our learning to greater depths than other faculty members in our health fields were able to provide. In his own animated way, he would pound his fists against his chest and ask, "Can you see that?" He was referring to that self-esteem growing within us. He insisted that who we are today is as good as who we were yesterday, and is as good as who we will be tomorrow.

Kekuni truly connected with each of us. And he helped us connect our learning with what we were actually doing for our people. He took the time to honor these connections because he was a lifelong learner alongside us.

Expanding Theory of Kānaka Maoli Health Change

Those of us in the health profession benefited greatly from Kekuni's unique mentoring style, strong cultural identity, and profound knowledge. Though

Kekuni was an expert in the specialized fields of hematology and pathology, he looked at the bigger picture of what causes disease to occur, not just the biological factors. He taught us how to adapt typical medical models so that we could quickly grasp the cultural and historical context of the health of our people.

Kekuni was steadfast in teaching that for Kānaka Maoli to heal today, we need to address our sociopolitical history. He was at the forefront of publishing and promoting the wealth of knowledge our kāhuna held, and he was able to articulate—in clear terms that all of us could understand—why our traditional system of ola flourished for generations before foreign influence modified our distinctive philosophy of care.

Beyond being a world-class physician when there were but a few Native Hawaiian medical doctors we could look to, Kekuni was an accomplished scholar. He took time to patiently study Hawaiian history, anthropology, and ʻōlelo Hawaiʻi. Never relying solely on Western medicine, Kekuni was an advocate for traditional Hawaiian medicine and was able to effectively document that perspective for supporters and critics alike. He had the ability to look at cultural remedies to solve present-day problems—something even more remarkable when considering that Kekuni was the first chair of medicine at the John A. Burns School of Medicine at the University of Hawaiʻi, where he studied with and built upon the work of greats such as Ozzie Bushnell.

Kekuni wrote the health section of the Native Hawaiians Study Commission report in June 1983, which was produced and funded by the Office of Hawaiian Affairs. This landmark report documented health issues and convened critical conversations to theorizing health promotion among Kānaka—for instance, why having more Kānaka in health fields was paramount to improving the quality and longevity of life for our people in a concrete way. He then took that research, created programs, and changed policies to activate the findings of the report.

Examining the effects of colonized conditions such as alcohol abuse, infectious disease, and unhealthy behaviors was a part of our methodology, but Kekuni talked about interventions through the lens of a cultural remedy first. As a writer he was fluent in weaving in the importance of healthy diet, strong social ties, and clean and sanitary environments, which became celebrated themes in his work targeting the strength and resilience of the precontact traditional Hawaiian health system. Kekuni effortlessly related today's health sciences to the ʻoihana of our kūpuna: psychology and social work to ho'oponopono; medicine and pharmacy to lā'au lapa'au; nutrition and dietetics to 'ai pono; and physical therapy and chiropractic to lomilomi.

He integrated a maoli model of what health looks like for contemporary Hawaiians. We cannot refer to this integrated model without emphasizing that Kekuni made it okay to relate Hawaiian spirituality to healthy Hawaiians. He promoted a deep sense of cultural understanding and application of our values in the present day. Always willing to talk about past events that caused suffering to Kānaka Maoli, he was never embarrassed about post-colonial conditions we were trying to overcome in the 1980s and 1990s.

Kekuni understood that health disparities are not the result of isolated causes. For example, a person is not obese simply because they don't exercise. Rather, disease is inextricably linked to not having a home, or coming from an unsupportive family environment, or not having access to higher education to learn new skills—all of which are linked to historical events such as the illegal overthrow of our kingdom and the spiral away from who we are as a people, right here in our homeland. Following this logic, the remedy always traces back to actively healing us as a people. Kekuni understood these cultural determinants of health and was unrelenting in pointing us toward holistic solutions.

It is important to note that in the 1980s, there were real taboos in the medical and health sciences with regard to integrating religion, spirituality, culture, and ethnicity. But for Kekuni, these were all part of the equation. For example, he saw the associations and causal effects of diabetes, and he knew where we needed to build community interventions. Another example is how he could relate the 1819 abolition of the kapu system to the disintegration of our system of mauli ola (health and well-being). He would clearly trace the points in time that marked a shift away from prevention and maintenance of our healthy identity—physically, emotionally, mentally, economically, politically, and spiritually—toward a focus on the treatment of acute and chronic conditions. It was clear to Kekuni that without a guiding framework based on strong cultural and spiritual traditions, Hawaiians become systemically vulnerable to Western influence and effect. He never lost sight of our need and our ability to reconnect to that heritage of strength and wellness.

Although Kekuni was a rigorous academic, he shunned institutionalization and was never an "ivory tower" stereotype. He broke down silos through his practice, his programs, and his policies. He urged cross-disciplinary conversations and collaboration long before organizations and businesses began teaching them as best practices. To us, he did not define himself as a doctor but as a Kanaka who served the best interests of our lāhui. He embodied strong leadership and mirrored those values to us. This was evident decades ago when some of us were brought together to meet with Kekuni and Marjorie Mau at the Queen's Medical Center to discuss the early formation of the Department of Native Hawaiian Health at the John A. Burns School of Medicine. Now, many years later, we are witness to the abundance of Kānaka success stimulated by those conversations. That effort then, those small conversations, led to Hawaiʻi's only medical school dedicating a department to our people and our health. This is a powerful reminder of the impact of collective efforts.

Kekuni was future oriented but always grounded in our traditional Kanaka perspectives of mind, body, and spiritual connections. He saw the past as a framework to guide our future potential and to carry us beyond present-day health disparities. This is one of the most important lessons Kekuni's legacy has left for today and for the next generation.

Political Advocacy

Using his wisdom and position to protect Native Hawaiian health as an inherent right, Kekuni embodied true political diplomacy. He was never afraid to speak up, and he always did so with respect and aloha. Political science became a passion for him. It was more than general awareness or supplemental education—he applied his learning and became politically savvy.

Throughout his advocacy work, Kekuni emphasized lōkahi (unity) and the constant balancing of Kānaka with the akua and ʻāina. He reminded us that our relationships with one another, with the land, with the ocean, between Papa and Wākea, and even beyond our own shores are all part of being a healthy Hawaiian. He created a pathway for self-determination by weaving together science, community, and politics.

Kekuni's international relationships and esteem reached a global audience. In 1993 he convened Ka Hoʻokolokolonui Kānaka Maoli (The Peoples' International Tribunal, Hawaiʻi) during the centennial commemoration of the illegal overthrow of Queen Liliʻuokalani. He brought together Kānaka Maoli, Pacific Islanders, Polynesians, Puerto Ricans, and others to form deeper connections and to examine the past injustices of the United States and the state of Hawaiʻi. Twenty-five years later, Kekuni's influence is still felt as those involved in the tribunal continue their advocacy work in the broader arena of Indigenous peoples.

Advocacy came naturally to Kekuni. For example, at the 1998 Ka ʻUhane Lōkahi gathering at Kapiʻolani Community College, Kekuni led a breakout group on "ceded lands" and those ʻāina illegally seized from our kingdom. While facilitating the dialogue among health practitioners and providers, Kekuni asserted that we must systematically investigate the return of our ʻāina and the settlement of the public land trust. He suggested that by addressing the ʻāina, we would also be addressing the systemic health of our people. He understood that conditions of mauli ola are natural to this ʻāina, but that a significant reconciliation needed to occur so that our people and resources can once again thrive. Kekuni had an internal template in his mind of how to plant seeds of inquiry to advance critical conversations and advocate for forward movement of the lāhui.

Nurturing Pilina

Kekuni's successes did not come without scars. The work was challenging, so it was important to construct a strong foundation of pilina early on. Each time we would attend a gathering with Kekuni, he would connect us with others who were doing work of critical importance. He would say, "Do you know so-and-so mā? This is what they do." He would then walk us over to the person, make a personal introduction, and create a bridge that connected us from him to them. Every hoʻolauna (introduction) included a vocal intonation to stay alert, suggesting it was an important pilina Kekuni was opening for us. We viewed this as Kānaka building the network for lāhui growth, and we followed Kekuni's lead in connecting with other agents of change who were overcoming similar challenges.

From his personal and professional experiences—as well as his higher level of consciousness—Kekuni knew that the empowerment of Native Hawaiians is critical to our future identity and our healing process. He knew there is a political path to reconcile that truth with the state of Hawaiʻi, the United States, and international bodies. It was his way of not being afraid to take on the injustices that he understood at such a high level. While mentoring, we understood that you cannot do lāhui-level work alone, and that each of us plays a role in anchoring our purpose with kuleana and putting it into action. We were not begging for solutions for our well-being from outsiders then, and we will not do so now. We shouldn't have to. This is our ʻāina, our home, and this is our kuleana to uphold. That offends some people today, as it did in years past. But we have been entrusted to steward Kekuni's vision for its decision-making capacity and continue this collective effort in our respective capacities. Kekuni was courageous, and this gave all of us more courage to overcome difficulties that arose.

Kekuni did not pursue just one area of expertise. He took on primary care, tertiary care, acute care, and preventive care, and he excelled in all of them. He demonstrated that we can—and must—use a holistic approach in our practice. As his practice evolved over the years, Kekuni was a model for getting involved and staying involved. There were times when he would teach, then attend a protest, then participate in an ʻawa ceremony, and then sit down with us for a lunch of poi and laulau. He seemed to be able to accomplish more in a morning than most of us could do in a week. And even with all he was involved in, and all the obstacles he faced in upholding this sometimes heavy work, Kekuni was always warm, positive, and welcoming. That was who he was.

Remaining Inclusive

Kekuni was inclusive. He welcomed everyone. And he taught us how to be inclusive within our own vision for helping Kānaka mobilize without borders. This moved us toward the goal of social welfare for Hawaiʻi in the 1990s, with a focus on quality of life for Kānaka and the well-being of the entire lāhui.

We can recall many lively gatherings at Kekuni's home in Nuʻuanu in which we discussed health equity and social justice. But we knew we couldn't achieve these goals as singular hale—it would have to be done as kauhale (group of houses comprising a Hawaiian home). Kekuni used this image to move our learning into action as we transitioned roles over the years. This laid the foundation of responsibility for what we now maintain as contemporary Hawaiian health leaders who still ask the question of one another: how do we bring our people together, capture that mana, and move it forward for positive change? For us, moving from hale to kauhale is a metaphor for our collective potential and confidence to make positive change a reality.

Today, Kekuni's legacy continues to exert pressure on our public institutions. Has the state recognized the influence Kānaka Maoli have on the government when we come together? Has the University of Hawaiʻi recognized the influence Kānaka Maoli have on the educational system as an Indigenous-serving institution? These questions can be answered in many ways, but one thing is certain: Kekuni's insistence on inclusivity has led to the state and university being increasingly responsible to our community.

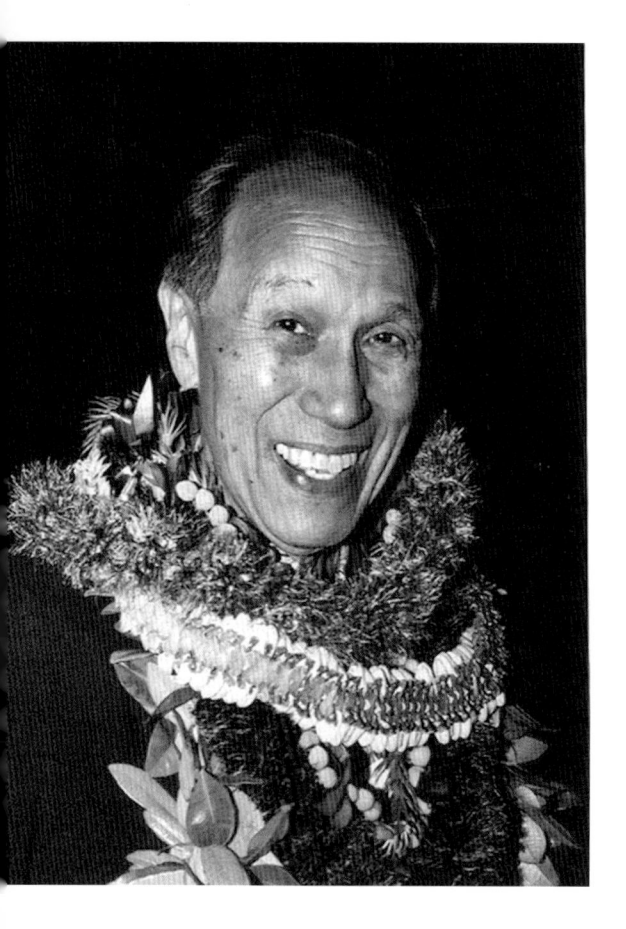

Kekuni genuinely wanted Kānaka Maoli to be leaders across organizations, to speak of historical injustice, to share our vision of health and well-being, to influence change, to be at the table, to make decisions that benefit our people, and to hold others accountable in their positions that affect Hawaiians and our homeland. Central to all of Kekuni's teachings was the goal for us to systemically advocate across sectors, within multiple levels, and across disciplines. He knew that if we became Kanaka leaders of high-impact organizations, with this type of integrated training, that we could also become advocates and not have to rely on others to speak on our behalf. It was truly a privilege to learn leadership skills from someone who was right there, truly leading.

Kekuni did not always have a goal of achievement for himself. Instead, he valued the developmental process by including haumāna in his own growth. Those personal traits of inclusion never changed and never wavered in Kekuni's commitment to execute lāhui goals.

Closing Recommendation

Kekuni was an integral catalyst for change spanning three generations. We can look back, reflect on his teachings, remember his actions, and restore our lāhui through the role we ʻauamo (pole or stick used for carrying burdens across the shoulders) today. We close these personal reflections with a recommendation pursuant to Kekuni's values and expectations of Kānaka Maoli health leaders striving to benefit the Hawaiian community.

We recommend creating an Institute of Kānaka Maoli Health and Wellness that convenes the masses to carry Kekuni's vision forward for another three generations. We envision a transdisciplinary institute led by Kānaka as a venue for collaboration to continue mauli ola loa (enduring health and well-being). We imagine culturally centered care as foundational to the institute's mission, with those who practice this ideology becoming experts and leading change for the long-term health and success of our lāhui. We predict that this institute will propel Kanaka well-being and eliminate Native Hawaiian health disparities by the year 2100. We foresee ʻōhiʻa groves that mature despite rough barriers, and lehua blossoming with pride in the face of harsh conditions.

Kekuni truly believed that his vision of culturally centered care could be translated into a reality. Thanks to the foundation he set for us, it is within our capability to dedicate a physical space and begin cultivating the necessary relationships to make this happen.

For his entire life, Kekuni was a master of crossing boundaries. Now that he has crossed from this life to the next, we look forward to his continued spiritual guidance to lead us forward for many years to come. With fond aloha we remember his Kanaka heart and hold fast to these famous words:

Hū wale aʻe nā hoʻomanaʻo ʻana	*Memories come*
Nō nā aliʻi kaulana	*Of the famous chiefs,*
Ua pau, ua hala lākou	*They are gone, they have passed,*
A koe nō nā pua.	*And their flowers survive.*

(Samuel Kuahiwi in Elbert
and Mahoe 1970, 79–80)

This chapter was originally published as "Kū ka ʻŌhiʻa i ka ʻAʻā—ʻŌhiʻa That Stands amid the Lava Fields," in *Hūlili: Multidisciplinary Research on Hawaiian Well-Being* 11, no. 2 (2019): 323–338. Reprinted here with permission. Photos of Kekuni Blaisdell by Deborah Dimaya.

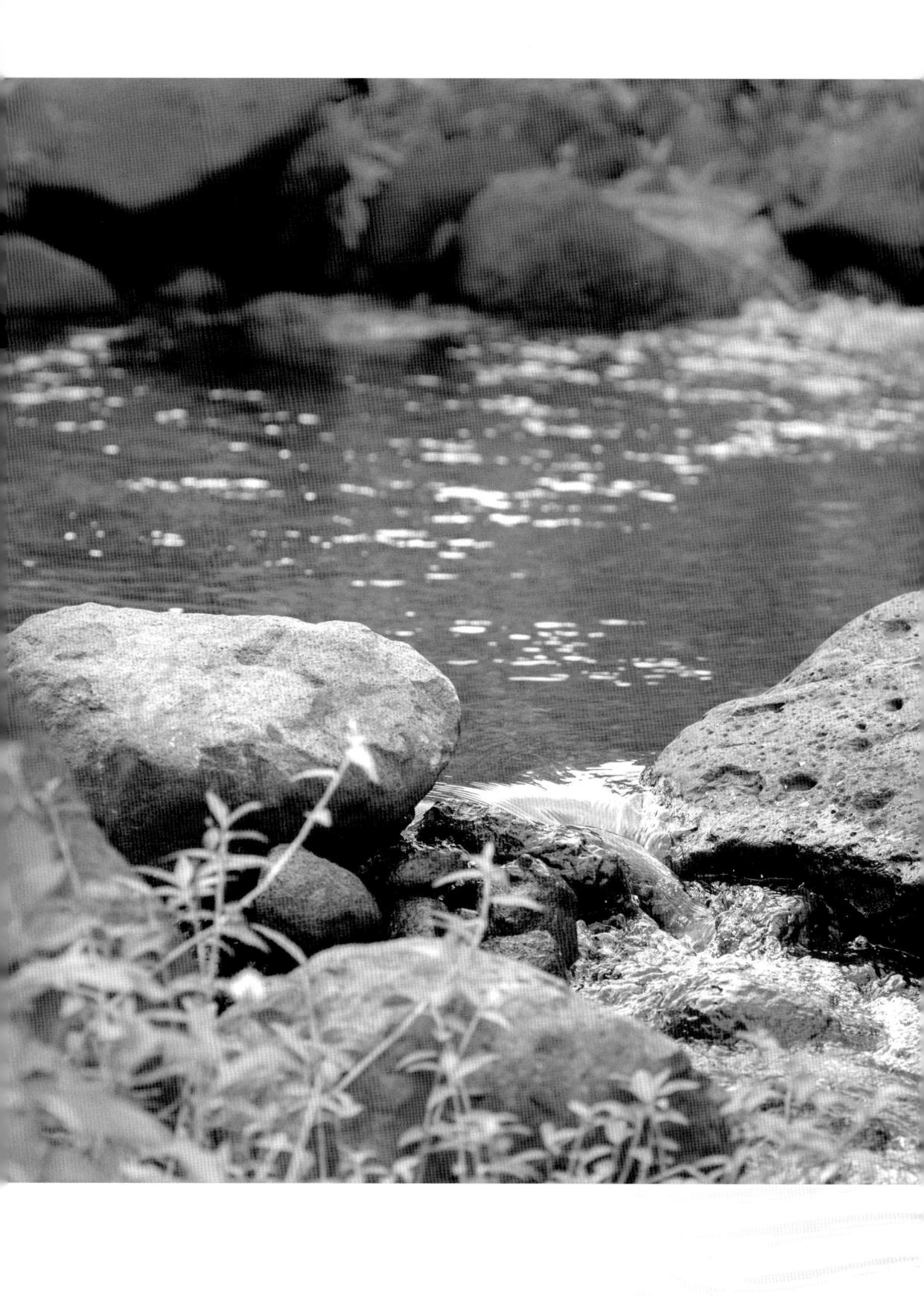

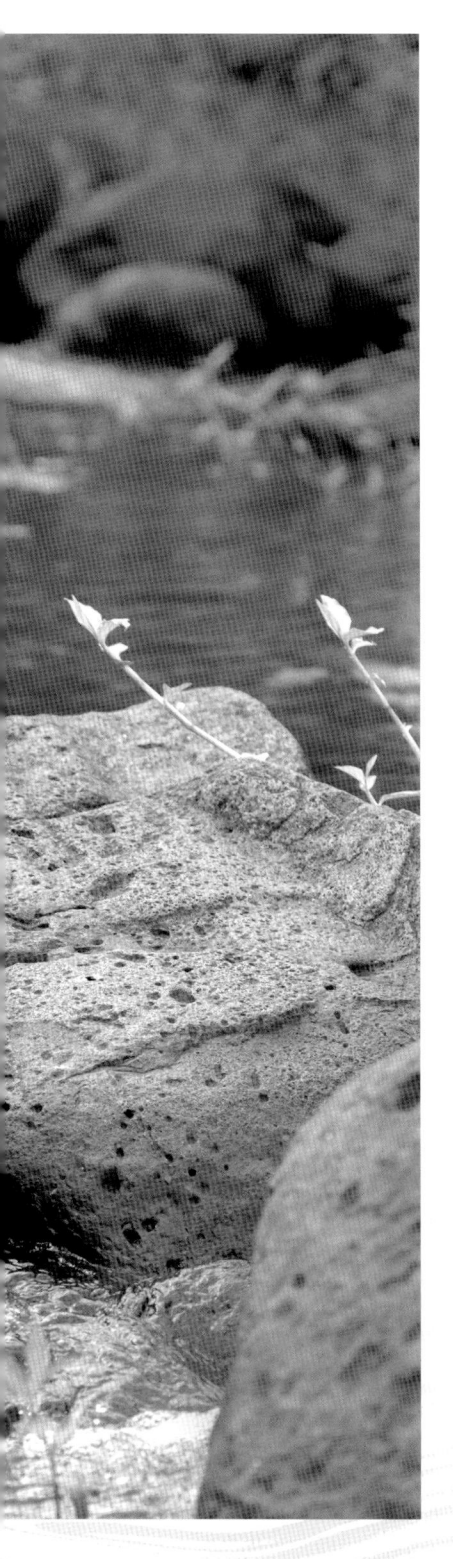

CHAPTER 16

Hoʻopau

As conveyed in the title of this book, *Ka Māno Wai: The Source of Life,* we view ancestral practices as a source of life that is symbolically represented by fresh water. As an essential natural resource, water is central to Hawaiian cosmology, in which there is emphasis on the spiritual foundation and interconnectedness of all things. Kāne, a Hawaiian God who is recognized as giving life to humankind and Earth (Kanahele 1986), is physically represented by water. Its life sustaining properties circulate through the system, nourishing people and the environment. Similarly, ancestral practices sustain life by circulating as the foundation of culture and affirming the linkages of the past, present, and future. Ancestral practices preserve culture and hold answers for health and social justice today.

The kumu loea who shared their stories in this book are treasured resources who keep ancestral practices vibrant and relevant for contemporary life. They are knowledge keepers of Hawaiian culture, master practitioners, and esteemed teachers. Each kumu loea is:

Ka waihona o ka naʻauao.

The repository of learning.

(Pukui 1983, 178)

The urgency in capturing the wisdom of these knowledge keepers is best reflected in a statement from ʻŌlohe lua Jerry Walker: "It has been said that every time an elder dies, you lose a library."

Underlying kumu loea stories are three intersecting and fundamental principles. First, the promotion of ancestral practices of Kānaka provides linkages between the past, present, and future. Second, these linkages in the continuum of time are vital to the preservation of culture. Third, Kānaka ancestral practices provide the possibility and promise of improving health and social justice for Native Hawaiians and others.

As you engaged with these stories, a number of common themes across kumu loea should have emerged. For example, kumu loea attended to the pilina of spirituality, environment, and people associated with the origins and practices of their specialty areas. Mana is inherent in practices guided by spiritual standards, and mana has transformative value when infused and shared by kumu loea in practices that deal with health and social justice. Kumu loea maintained the authenticity of ancestral practices while making modifications for the current context of Hawaiʻi and Hawaiians. Kumu loea attributed importance to the sense of place, and place shaped their development as practitioners. They collectively viewed genealogy and family as central to their identity and growth. They understood that the use of ʻōlelo Hawaiʻi is necessary for a foundational understanding of Hawaiian ways of knowing, thinking, and being. Lastly, all kumu loea demonstrated a humility about their expertise, attributing their skills to akua, their family, their kumu, their colleagues, and their haumāna.

Sources of Knowledge for Kumu Loea

The inspiration from kumu loea becomes more profound as we begin to better understand the lineage of knowledge in regard to who taught them and how they learned. In telling their stories, kumu loea are clear on their kuleana in perpetuating culture. They simultaneously acknowledge their appreciation for their sources of ʻike.

The training and education of kumu loea in their distinctive areas came primarily from three sources: (a) family, (b) cultural experts, and (c) historical and contemporary cultural writings. In learning from these sources, kumu loea were explicit about the diversity and richness of knowledge and would remind us that their approach "represents only one way of doing this" or "may be different from other people" or "was the way I was taught by my kumu." The fundamental importance is that training and education were rooted in the honoring of cultural values. The following sections highlight sources of knowledge.

Family Foundations

Kumu loea attributed their foundation of cultural learning to early teaching and training that began at home, with family. The influence of family in one's training has roots in ancestral learning. In old Hawaiʻi, children received their education through listening, observing, and taking part in daily life. "In the Hawaiian ʻohana, the extended family of the past, the young child began to watch, listen, and therefore, learn, long before parents or grandparents began any planned instruction" (Pukui et al. 1979, 49). The important influence of family also is expressed in this ʻōlelo noʻeau:

KA ʻIKE A KA MAKUA HE HEI NA KE KEIKI.

The knowledge of the parent is [unconsciously] absorbed by the child.

(PUKUI 1983, 151)

As children, kumu loea learned through their relationships with their family, nature, and the spiritual realm. They learned by listening to and observing and modeling behaviors of family members as they engaged in healing, land cultivation, and ocean dynamics. Many learned cultural protocol, practices, and principles through daily living activities, while some were intentionally trained in particular areas. All rely on the transmission of cultural knowledge from one generation to the next to ensure its perpetuation. For example, Lynette Paglinawan describes being reared in a family of healers who provided an abundance of learning opportunities. Hoʻoponopono was integrated into family life, and Lynette learned quickly about its importance in maintaining familial relationships. Understanding the critical role of family harmony in the survival (physical, emotional, and spiritual) of the family and culture became fundamental hallmarks in her work in hoʻoponopono.

Sarah Keahi spoke fondly of her childhood and learning from her kūpuna. In particular, Sarah often found herself sitting with her grandmother and her friends listening intently to their conversations in ʻōlelo Hawaiʻi. She vividly recalls how each word effortlessly rolled off their tongues, and when strung together, created a lei of sounds that were like the beautiful melodies of the forest birds. These observations of everyday activities at home with her family provided the foundation for Sarahʻs passion in teaching Hawaiian language.

Eric Enos' love and appreciation for the ʻāina is rooted in the childhood memories of growing up with his family in Mākaha. Eric recalls spending time with his parents, who taught him skills in farming, irrigation, and building. He also recalls spending time sewing lei from the flowers they grew at their home. These activities helped instill in Eric a deep love of the ʻāina, which remains the driving force behind his advocacy efforts to create ʻāina momona in communities across Hawaiʻi.

Many cultural practices employ disciplined processes and protocols that typically start with observation, and include deeper training and practice. For example, Kamanaʻopono Crabbe describes his childhood as growing up in two worlds, Western and Hawaiian, with his family lifestyle being characterized as very Hawaiian. Having ample opportunity to participate in everyday activities such as fishing, crabbing, and picking ʻopihi, Kamanaʻopono developed a sense of honor and pride for mea Hawaiʻi. This, along with spending lots of time with his granduncle learning about moʻokūʻauhau, set him on a path toward understanding, articulating, and teaching about mana.

Holding the role of punahele, Kaleo Paik was explicitly chosen by her father to learn the formidable family practice of helping loved ones pass from life to death. Kaleo recounts learning from her father as she accompanied him to offer his earnest comfort to families in grief and bereavement. This, along with formal training and practice, ultimately contributed to her style and form of mālama kūpuna with an emphasis on caring for Hawaiian iwi, and supporting people in the transition from life to death.

Leinaʻala Bright warmly recalls her childhood in California, where her family honored and lived the Hawaiian culture, sharing values, moʻolelo, mele, hula, healing, and pule. With that as her foundation, she began to develop a deeper connection to lomilomi and lāʻau lapaʻau. Early familial observations and teaching are the cornerstone of her cultural reverence and respect, from which she is able to thrive as a Native Hawaiian healer and practitioner.

While the family provides a foundation for learning ancestral practices, genealogical information can further fortify efforts to learn about culture. For example, Melody MacKenzie learned from her grandmother that she carries one of the names of Princess Miriam Likelike. Growing up, Melody heard many mo‘olelo about the service of her great-grandfather to King Kalākaua and Queen Lili‘uokalani, affirming the family's historical and cultural linkages to the Hawaiian community. These stories strengthened her kuleana and inspired her commitment to social justice, and, specifically, Native Hawaiian law.

As in old Hawai‘i, education for our kumu loea did not end with their participation in family life and daily activities. They also intentionally pursued education in specialty areas from experts and learning "specific things under competent instruction" (Handy et al. 1965, 59).

Cultural Experts

Cultural experts are a vital source of education and training in Hawaiian culture. Kumu loea who identified a cultural expert as their kumu recognized this person as pivotal to their experience of Kānaka culture and the learning of specialty areas. These experts are renowned in their areas and held a special teacher-student relationship with the kumu loea featured in this book. In some ways, education by cultural experts broadly resembled the apprenticeship model evident in Hawai‘i long ago: "There was instruction by experts. It was sound and excellent instruction, for it was really apprenticeship. Apprenticeship means that the young person takes part in the work, learns under an expert, and works on the job until he has mastered the skills and crafts involved. This is much more effective training than school instruction. Education in old Hawai‘i was very practical and effective" (Handy et al. 1965, 55).

One similarity between the apprenticeship model and the way kumu loea learn today emphasizes mastering skills in practical ways. Several kumu loea were trained by experts associated with a culture-based school. Examples of this type of learning include lua and ho‘oponopono. Jerry Walker's lua teacher was the distinguished ‘Ōlohe Charles Kenn, whose elite style of training is linked to Kamehameha I. From this educational lineage, Jerry, along with four other lua masters, established premier schools of lua, Pā Ku‘i-a-Lua and Pā Ku‘i-a-Holo. Two other featured kumu loea, ‘Umi Kai and Sonny Kaulukukui, achieved the status of ‘ōlohe in these schools. "To become an ‘Ōlohe in the past would have required twenty years of study. Today, both schools have graduated ‘Ōlohe in four to nine years" (Paglinawan et al. 2006, 30). Training in lua provided the impetus for ‘Umi in his work with nā mea kaua and Sonny in his work with kaula and Hawaiian weaponry.

Lynette Paglinawan acknowledges many experts in hoʻoponopono and recognizes that many families had their own styles of hoʻoponopono. She consistently speaks of her training by noted historian, scholar, and practitioner Mary Kawena Pukui, who influenced generations of students with her approach to hoʻoponopono. In the third volume of *Nānā I Ke Kumu* (2020), coauthored by Lynette and Richard Likeke Paglinawan, Dennis Kauahi, and Valli Kalei Kanuha, hoʻoponopono is described as the style that "follows the spirit and teaching of Tūtū Pukui and Auntie Malia Craver" (p. 77). While Lynette recognizes that hoʻoponopono may have been modified over the years, the process, cultural values, and basic elements are the same as those taught her.

Several kumu loea were significantly affected by cultural experts they knew for many years. For example, Sarah Keahi speaks fondly of the guidance of Dr. Samuel H. Elbert, a linguist and professor emeritus at the University of Hawaiʻi at Mānoa (UHM). Along with Mary Kawena Pukui, Dr. Elbert authored the seminal *Hawaiian Dictionary* (1986), which has helped people with Hawaiian and English translations. In a conversation with Dr. Elbert, Sarah accepted her kuleana to become a teacher of ʻōlelo Hawaiʻi.

Dr. Claire Hughes has worked for decades to promote healthy eating, and she acknowledges Dr. Kekuni Blaisdell, a physician, scholar and activist, as a longtime mentor and friend. The two of them worked together in the 1980s, along with Dr. Emmett Aluli, to establish the nutritional composition of the traditional Hawaiian diet. The team then went on to test the diet and found that it reduced cholesterol and blood glucose levels in overweight participants on Molokaʻi. In addition to an appreciation for scientific testing, Claire admired Kekuni for this facility of crafting Hawaiian-language names for health-oriented groups. An example is the name Hoʻoulu (to grow, sprout, propagate; to cause to increase), which he bestowed on a group dedicated to spreading the word about and expanding the impact of the traditional Hawaiian diet.

Jon Osorio's parents grounded him in mele with ʻukulele lessons from Kumu Danby Beamer and singing in church. But Jon was especially influenced by George Helm, a Hawaiian musician and legendary activist of the aloha ʻāina movement. Jon admired Helm's ability to intricately weave stories about the circumstances of the Hawaiian people and to use mele to educate and inspire others in social advocacy and justice. Jon also appreciated Helm's deep understanding of the songs he sang, which encouraged Jon to further his knowledge of ʻōlelo Hawaiʻi and the kaona of Hawaiian words and phrases.

It is not uncommon for kumu loea to have received training from several cultural experts in different specialty areas. Kumu loea showed themselves to be lifelong learners of Hawaiian culture, as they availed themselves of learning from cultural experts in related but diverse areas. For example, Keola Chan learned Auntie Margaret Machado's style of lomilomi from Sheila O'Malley, a student of Auntie Margaret who was given permission to teach. With this anchoring in lomilomi, Keola also studied with other cultural experts, including Auntie Malia Craver in hoʻoponopono and with Auntie Alapaʻi Kahuʻena in lāʻau lapaʻau.

Similarly, Dr. Kamanaʻopono Crabbe credits many mentors and role models for his education, including Kumu Hokulani Holt-Padilla, Auntie Abbie Napeahi, Auntie Malia Craver, Earl Kawaʻa, Richard Likeke Paglinawan, Billy Kahalepuna Richards, Gordon ʻUmi Kai, and others. In line with his approach to mana, Kamanaʻo believes that training in ritual ceremony, hoʻoponopono, and lua can enhance the acquisition of mana for teacher and student.

Leinaʻala Bright also recognizes many cultural influences in her education as she espouses an integrated style of practice, including lāʻau lapaʻau, lomilomi, and pule. She credits Kumu Levon Ohai for her training in lāʻau lapaʻau, noting that Ohai's lineage of learning goes back several generations, and she acknowledges Kumu Alva Andrews for her training in a school of lomilomi that can be traced through the Peʻa family for over five hundred years. She also studied hula with Kumu John Kahaʻi Topolinski and lua with ʻŌlohe Mitchell Eli and ʻŌlohe Jerry Walker.

Eric Enos also learned from many experts, including Donald Anderson, an expert in kalo; Dalani Tanahy Kauihou, an expert in making kapa; and Walter Paulo and Uncle Eddie Kaʻanana, experts in traditional fishing techniques. The knowledge amassed from these and other cultural experts, combined with knowledge gained through reading accounts of traditional land management practices, was compiled into a book *From Then to Now: A Manual for Doing Things Hawaiian Style* (Kaʻala Farm ʻOhana 1996). The book provides a practical guide for living in harmony with the land.

The prominence of education and training by family members and experts makes sense in Native Hawaiian culture, in which there was historical reliance on oral-aural communication. These learning interactions, based on listening, observing, and applying skills to real-life situations, served to transmit and preserve information. However, with the acquisition of reading and writing skills in the early to mid-1800s (Laimana 2011) and the publication of more than one hundred different Hawaiian-language nūpepa between 1834 and 1948 (Lorenzo-Elarco 2019), many kumu loea began to use cultural writings and university classes as additional sources of knowledge.

Historical and Contemporary Cultural Writings

Many kumu loea learned about their specialty areas by reading historical and contemporary documents and, in some cases, attending university classes and preparing their own documents for the further transmission of Hawaiian ʻike.

For example, Keola Chan spent countless hours diving into historical documents at the Bishop Museum archives, researching everything he could on lomilomi and the traditional Hawaiian structure of healing. He was especially guided by the book *Must We Wait in Despair: The 1867 Report of the ʻAhahui Lāʻau Lapaʻau of Wailuku, Maui on Native Hawaiian Health,* translated and edited by Malcolm Nāea Chun (1994).

ʻUmi Kai gained knowledge of nā mea kaua by researching historical documents by Te Rangi Hiroa (1957), Samuel Manaiakalani Kamakau (1964), and David Malo (1951). Te Rangi Hiroa, also known as Sir Peter Buck, was the first Western-trained anthropologist of Polynesian (Māori) ancestry, a world-renowned expert in Polynesian crafts, and director of the Bishop Museum from 1936 to 1951. His books, later compiled into a single volume, *Arts and Crafts of Hawaii,* provide rich descriptions of Hawaiian traditional objects, their uses, and their methods of construction (Hiroa 1957).

Sonny Kaulukukui also studied the works of David Malo and Samuel Kamakau. During his lifetime, Malo (1793–1853) was a chiefly counselor and a Hawaiian intellectual and educator. His books, written in ʻōlelo Hawaiʻi, document Hawaiian history and traditions. Kamakau (1815–1876) was a Hawaiian historian and scholar. His work appeared in local nūpepa, and much of it was later compiled into books. English translations of the writings of Malo and Kamakau were published by the Bishop Museum. Sonny also read botanical research reports by Isabella Abbott and Catherine Summers to support his work in kaula.

Jerry Walker's learning about lua was informed by his review of *ʻŌlelo Noʻeau Hawaiian Proverbs and Poetical Sayings* by Pukui (1983), through which he identified nearly one hundred proverbs on warriors and warfare. After studying lua with ʻŌlohe Charles Kenn, Jerry and colleagues decided to write a seminal book about lua, *Lua, Art of the Hawaiian Warrior* (Paglinawan et al. 2006). The book provides a tribute to ʻŌlohe Kenn and ensures that the basics of lua are never lost.

Kaleo Paik learned from her father to help individuals pass from life to death. However, in contemporary times, she has also been called to help with the reburial of iwi of Native Hawaiians found during the constructions of roads, housing, railway lines, and so forth. She has become very knowledgeable about the Native American Graves Protection and Repatriation Act (NAGPRA 1990) and other documents pertaining to the return of human remains and cultural objects excavated on tribal lands or belonging to poʻe kahiko. She has also become a documentarian herself, using poetry as a vehicle for articulating and communicating knowledge about the repatriation and interment of Native Hawaiian kūpuna iwi (Paik 2013) and about the preservation of legendary places in Hawaiʻi (Paik 2009).

Although much of Kamanaʻopono Crabbe's cultural learning was through the memorization of Hawaiian oli, including mele koʻihonua, he also studied ʻōlelo Hawaiʻi at Kapiʻolani Community College and earned master's and doctoral degrees in psychology at the UHM. Drawing on ʻike from the family and the university, Kamanaʻo and a team from the Office of Hawaiian Affairs worked on understanding the importance of mana. In addition to speaking with many Hawaiians, they researched the writings of Hawaiian scholars, ʻōlelo noʻeau, and nūpepa for usage of the word "mana." This research culminated in the publication of *Mana Lāhui Kānaka,* which provides a discourse that articulates the context and complexity of mana in Hawaiian culture (Crabbe, Fox, and Coleman 2017).

Melody MacKenzie gained insights into Hawaiian justice by reading historical documents, including the Kānāwai Māmalahoe, or Law of the Splintered Paddle, of 1797. This edict by Kamehameha I outlined rules for ensuring basic human rights. Melody also studied law at UHM and was mentored by William S. Richardson, a Native Hawaiian attorney who served as chief justice of the Hawaiʻi State Supreme Court (1966–1982). Combining knowledge and skills from these sources, she worked with colleagues to publish *Native Hawaiian Law: A Treatise.* This definitive book on critical legal issues for Native Hawaiians includes chapters on land and sovereignty, individual land titles, natural resource rights, traditional and customary rights, and resources for Native Hawaiians (MacKenzie, Serrano, and Sproat 2015).

Jon Osorio started to become familiar with ʻōlelo Hawaiʻi at home, at Kamehameha Schools, and through Hawaiian music. However, to really learn how to speak the language well enough to compose songs in ʻōlelo Hawaiʻi, he

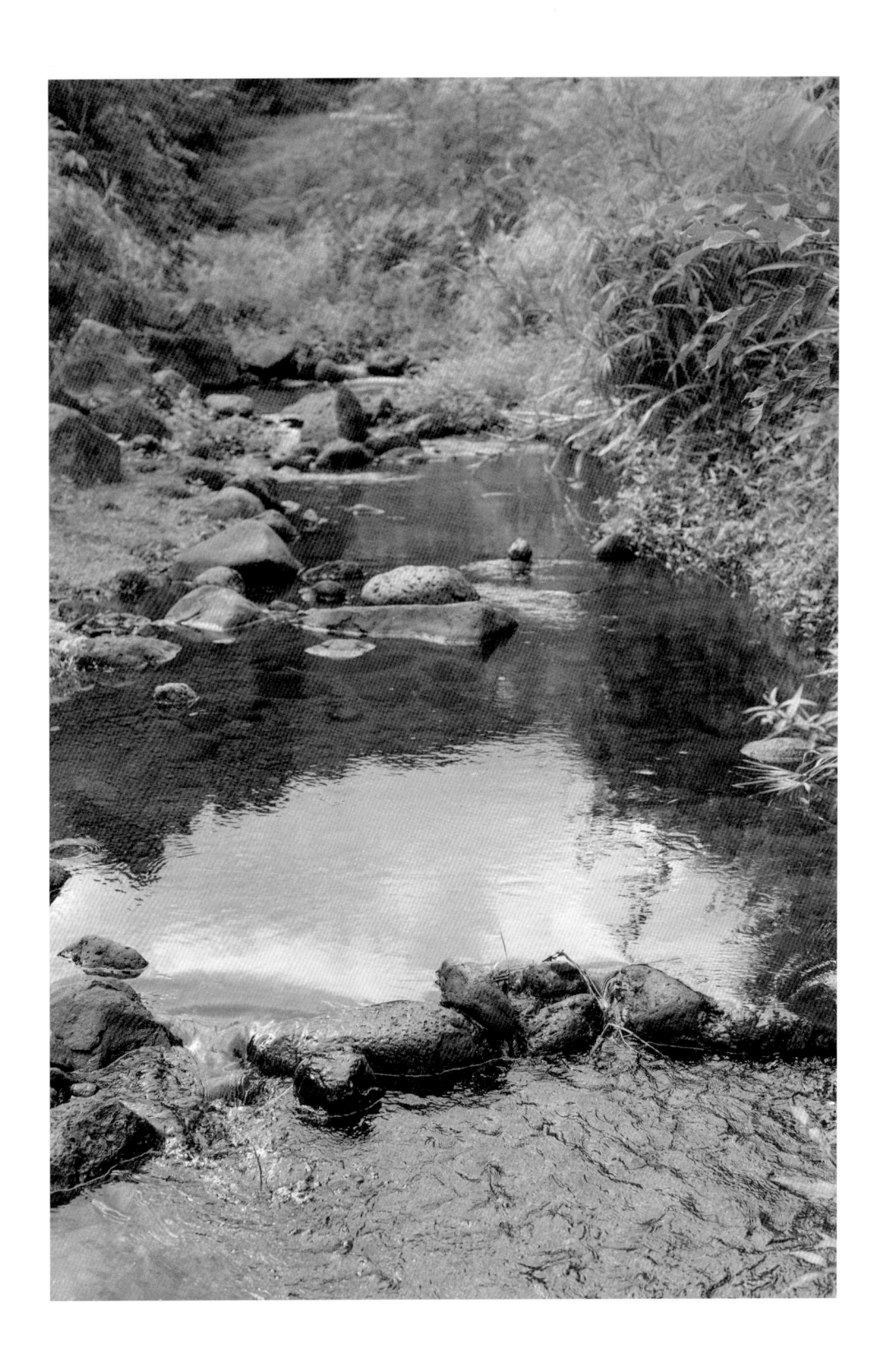

returned to the UHM to study the Hawaiian language. He later joined the faculty and is now dean of the Hawai'inuiākea School of Hawaiian Knowledge, which offers courses and degree programs in Hawaiian language and culture for students of all ages and walks of life. Although Jon Osorio has gained knowledge through his own research, which he has reported on in numerous chapters and books, he also learned through creating and helping others compose mele to express social, cultural, and political events and feelings. Two of his memorable songs reflecting justice and advocacy are *Hawaiian Eyes* and *Hawaiian Soul.*

Similarly, Claire Hughes returned to UHM to earn master's and doctoral degrees in public health. Although she was trained as a dietician in the continental United States, her doctoral studies focused on the traditional Hawaiian diet and its role in promoting health. Reviewing historical documents, Claire learned the first Western visitors to the islands found that "the Hawaiian people were splendid physical specimens and that their diet must have contained the elements necessary for health" (Handy et al. 1965, 95). Research skills gained through her university education allowed her to collaborate on the design of scientific studies that proved the significant health benefits of the traditional Hawaiian diet in reducing weight, blood pressure, blood sugar, and cholesterol. As longtime writer for a health column in *Ka Wai Ola,* the Office of Hawaiian Affairs newspaper, Claire continues to incorporate historical information on a variety of topics, including health, disease, nutrition, and lifestyle, to cultivate an appreciation of ancestral practices for contemporary life.

Panina (Closing)

Ka Māno Wai: The Source of Life is a compilation of mo'olelo of kumu loea who are authoritative experts on ancestral practices. Their stories demonstrate a building of expertise through personal development intertwined with training and education in specialty areas. As experts, they are always quick to acknowledge common sources of their own training and education, including family, cultural experts, and historical and contemporary cultural writings. In all learning experiences, there are explicit and implicit references to the importance of relationships, with special attention to spirituality.

Wai is one of the most important elements on Earth, and holds deep spiritual significance for Native Hawaiians, which perhaps explains the elevation of wai found not only in Hawai'i but throughout Polynesia as well.

Native Hawaiians have a "clear understanding that fresh water is the foundation of all life" (Sproat 2015, 525). When the word for "water" is repeated in ‘ōlelo Hawai‘i, its meaning is enhanced, and "waiwai is the Hawaiian word for wealth" (Kanahele 1986, 364). The cultural connotation of wealth is less about possessions and more about the sanctity and abundance of relationships.

The ancestral practices shared by kumu loea are like wai in being life-giving and in having deep grounding in the interrelation of Kānaka, akua, and ‘āina. In the mo‘olelo of kumu loea, we are reminded that Kānaka define life "by the quality of their relationships with family members, the community, the land, and the spiritual world" (Ewalt and Mokuau 1995). In this manner, ancestral practices are a source of cultural wealth that link generations—past, present, and future—with possible solutions for health and social justice.

Glossary

Definitions apply to usage in the book. For other definitions see Pukui and Elbert 1986.

'a'ali'i: native hardwood shrub
aho: cords
ahupua'a: land division
'ai: to eat, food
'ai kapu: system specifically regulated food and eating practices
'ai kūpele: therapeutic nutrition
'aiaola: to eat nutritious foods
'āina: land, to eat
'āina hānau: birthplace
'āina momona: fertile, fruitful land, and ocean
akua: gods
ali'i: chief, chiefs
ali'i wahine: women chiefs
aloha: love, affection, compassion
aloha 'āina: love for the land
aloha aku, aloha mai: aloha given, aloha received
anahulu: a period of ten days
'anakē: auntie
Ani: lua God
'anu'u tower: raised place
apu: traditional coconut serving cups
'auamo: pole or stick used for carrying burdens across the shoulders
'aumākua: ancestors, family gods
'auwai: water channels

'awa ceremony: a ceremony in which a drink from the kava plant is prepared, passed, and sipped as a sign of commitment to things Hawaiian
'awapuhi: ginger

calabash: bowl
chicken long rice: dish of chicken and rice or bean vermicelli noodles

e ala i hana no Kane: awake to work for Kane
e ho'okahua: make Kānaka Maoli strengths and resilience the foundation of our work
e ho'okāhuna: provide mentoring of Kānaka Maoli
e ho'okanaka: be a person of worth
e ho'okū: embrace the active use of Hawaiian values and practices
e ho'ōla: nurture leadership within the Kānaka community
e ho'omau ana kākou: let us persevere
e ho'oulu: build a collective vision that is forward-looking
'eha: pain, injury

hā: breath

ha he hu: guttural chorus of breathing

ha'awina 'ōlelo Hawai'i: Hawaiian language lessons

hāhā: palpation

hahano: cleansing

ha'i mo'olelo: storytelling

ha'iha'i iwi: bone setting

haku: braid or braided

haku hana no'eau: artist work

haku mele: to compose songs

hala: transgression; pandanus tree

hale: house

hale 'āina: women's eating house

hali'a aloha: cherished memory

Hāloa: son of Wākea

hana: work

hana lawelawe: serving chiefs

hānai: fostered, adopted

haole: Caucasian

haole koa: invasive species from the mimosoid tree family

hau: a type of hibiscus

haumāna: student, students

heiau: spiritual site

hemo: untie

hihia: entanglement of emotions, reactions, and interactions all in a negative way through acts of commission or omission

hili: braiding

hilo: first night of the new moon; twisting

hina: fall, topple, or lean over

Hina: Hawaiian God

hoa aloha: friends

hō'ailona: important sign and message from ancestors

ho'ēmi: to diminish

ho'i hou: seeking knowledge by turning to ancestral sources

hō'ike: presentation

hō'i'o: fern

Hōkūle'a: contemporary Hawaiian voyaging canoe

honi: traditional Hawaiian greeting exchanging breath, nose to nose

ho'ohanau keiki: baby-delivery

ho'ohāpai: induction of pregnancy

ho'okama: loved and treated as one's own

Ho'okē 'Ai: Moloka'i diet study

ho'okipa: hospitality

ho'olauna: introduction

ho'omaka: to begin, opening

ho'omalu: to make calm or to provide a period of silence

ho'omana: spirituality

ho'omau: perseverance, persistence

ho'onui: enlarge

ho'opau: to finish, finishing

ho'oponopono: setting to right, the process of conflict resolution

ho'oulu: to grow, sprout, propagate; to cause to increase

hua: fruit, fruitful

Hua: lua God

hula: dance

huli: turn over

huna: hidden, secret

i'a: fish

'ie'ie: aerial roots

ihe: short spear

ihu: nose

'ike: knowledge

'ike kūhohonu: deep knowledge

'ike kūpuna: ancestral knowledge

'ike lihilihi: close observation

imu: underground oven

ina kaua e Ku'i-a-lua: fight with me, Ku'i-a-lua

inoa: names
inoa kupuna: ancestral name
ipu: gourd
iwi: bones

kaʻane: strangling cord
kaʻao: legends
kahakai: coastal zone
kahawai: river; freshwater ecosystems, and streams
kāhea: call
kāhili: feather standard, feather standards, symbol of royalty
kahu hānai: adopted family
kahua: foundation
kahuna: expert
kāhuna: experts
kahuna moʻokūʻauhau: expert in genealogy
kahuna o na kiʻi: high priest
kai: salt water, ocean
kaka uhu: fishing with a decoy fish
kākoʻo: support
kala: untie, freeing, release
kālaimoku: chief counselor
kālika: garlic
kalo: taro
kamaliʻi: children
Kamapuaʻa: a pig demigod associated with the Hawaiian God Lono
Kanaka: Native Hawaiian
Kānaka: Native Hawaiians
kanaka kalaimoku or kālaimoku: chief counselor
Kānaka kāne: Hawaiian men
kānaka makua: enlightened, matured, and esteemed models of true Hawaiian character
Kānaka Maoli: Native Hawaiians
kānaka ʻōiwi: Native peoples
Kanaloa: Hawaiian God

kānāwai: laws
kānāwai akua: gods' laws
kānāwai kapu aliʻi: sacred chiefly laws
Kānāwai Māmalahoe: Law of the Splintered Paddle
Kāne: Hawaiian God
kāne: men
kāniwala: carnival
kānoa: ʻawa bowls
kanu: burial
kaona: hidden meaning
kapa: traditional Hawaiian cloth
kapa beater: tool to make cloth
kapu: taboo
kapu imu: an oven for preparing food for a ceremony
kapu system: code of conduct of standards and regulations
kauhale: group of houses comprising a Hawaiian home
kaula: cordage and rope
kaumaha: grief
kauwa: servants
Ke Akua: Christian God
keiki: child
keiki hānai: fostered or adopted child
kiaʻi: caretakers
Kihawahine: lua God
kīhei: cloak
kīhōʻalu: Hawaiian slack key
kilo: closely observe
kinolau: forms taken by a supernatural body
kīpuka: area of land ranging from several square meters to several square kilometers that supports plants and wildlife but is completely surrounded by lava
koa wāhine: brave women

koali: vine

koʻi: adzes

koʻihonua: genealogical chant

kōkō puʻupuʻu: intricately woven netting

kōkua: help

kolohe: wild, mischievous

Kū: Hawaiian God

kū: stand, upright, erect

Kū Kiaʻi Mauna: stand up for your mountain

kuʻi ʻakahi: first blow

kuʻi-a-holo: second blow

Kuʻi-a-holo: lua diety

Kuʻi-a-lua: principal deity of lua, second blow

kūkākūkā: discuss

kukui: candlenut tree

kūkulu hou: rebuilding

kūkulu kumuhana: statement of the problem

kuleana: responsibility, privilege

kumu: teacher

kumu hula: teacher of hula

kumu loea: expert teachers

kumu niu: coconut trees

kumu ʻōlelo Hawaiʻi: Hawaiian language teacher

kupuna: elder

kūpuna: elders, ancestors

kūpuna iwi: ancestral bones

kupuna wahine: grandmother

Kūwaha-ilo: lua deity

lāʻau: plant, medicine

lāʻau kāhea: a type of faith healing

lāʻau lapaʻau: Hawaiian medicinal plants

lāʻau pālau: long club

lāhui: Hawaiian nation

lau hala: pandanus leaf

Lauhau: lua God

laukahi: plantain

laulau: packages of ti leaves or banana leaves containing pork, beef, salted fish, or taro tops, baked in the ground oven, steamed or broiled

lei: garland

leina-a-ke-akua: place from which spirits leaped into eternity

leiomano: shark's teeth weapon

limu kala: seaweed

loʻi: irrigated taro terrace

lōkahi: unity

lokomaikaʻi: generosity

lomi: to rub, press, squeeze, crush, mash, knead, massage, rub out

lomi ʻaʻe: to massage the back with the feet

lomi salmon: dish made from salted salmon, tomatoes, onions, and green onions

lomilomi: to rub, press, knead, massage

Lono: Hawaiian God

Lonopūhā: first student of Kamakanuiʻāhaʻilono, God of healing

Lowahine: lua God

lua: Hawaiian art of fighting

lua ʻai: lua techniques

lūʻau: Hawaiian feast, Hawaiian feasts

mā: and others

maʻa: sling

mahele: division

mahiki: handling one problem at a time

mahiole: feather helmet

makaʻāinana: commoners, populace

Makahiki: a time of thanksgiving and ceremonial competition

makai: ocean side
Makaliʻi: Pleiades
makua: adult
māla: garden
mālama: care for
mālama ʻāina: care for the land
mālama iwi: care for ancestral bones
mālama kūpuna: care for elders and ancestors
malihini: tourists
malo: traditional Hawaiian loincloth
mana: spiritual, supernatural, or divine power
mana akua: mana from the gods
manini: small, trivial
maoli: native, indigenous
mauka: mountain side
mauli ola: health and well-being
mauli ola loa: enduring health and well-being
mauna: mountain, watershed
me ke aloha: with aloha
me ka mahalo nui: with much thankfulness
me ka mahalo palena ʻole: with gratitude beyond measure
me ka mahalo piha: with whole-hearted thankfulness
mea Hawaiʻi: Hawaiian things
mele: song, songs
Mele a Pākui: chant of the ancient gods and lineages of early chiefs in Hawaiʻi
mele koʻihonua: cosmogonic genealogical chants
mihi: to repent and forgive
moa: chicken
mōʻaukala: history
mōhalu: open or unfold like a flower
mōʻī: monarch
moku: district, place, island

momona: fat, fertile, plump, rounded, or sweet
moʻokūʻauhau: genealogy
moʻolelo: story, stories
moʻomeheu: culture
mua: men's house
muku: last moon of the thirty-day moon cycle

na hana imua: future tasks
nā mea kaua: Hawaiian weapons
nā piko ʻekolu: three body points
nā pule kahiko: ancient Hawaiian prayers
naʻau: mind, heart, or gut
nalu: ocean waves and surf
nānā: to closely observe
newa: short club
nīoi: Hawaiian chili pepper
niu: coconut
noni: Indian mulberry
nounou: field stones
nūpepa: newspapers

ʻohana: family
ʻohe kapala: bamboo stamps
ʻōhiʻa: tree that sprouts forth in the fresh lava field
oiaʻiʻo: truth, sincerity
ʻoihana: customs, activities
ʻoki: cut
ola: health
ʻōlelo: language
ʻōlelo Hawaiʻi: Hawaiian language
ʻōlelo nane: riddles, parables, allegories
ʻōlelo noʻeau: Hawaiian proverbs and poetical sayings, Hawaiian proverb and poetical saying
ʻōlelo pāpā: verbally challenge
ʻōlena: turmeric
oli: chant

'ōlohe: master teacher

'ōlohe koa: master warrior

'ōlohe lua: lua master

olonā: Native shrub

'ō'ō: bloodletting; pointed digging stick

'o'opu: fresh-water fish

'opelu: mackerel scad

'opihi: limpet

ōwī: blue vervain

pā: wall

pa'a: firm

pa'a kai: salt

pae 'āina: archipelago

pāhoa: dagger

pahu: drum

pakalana: Chinese violet

pani: closing ritual

panina: closing

Papa: ancestor of the Hawaiian people

papa ku'i 'ai: board on which poi is pounded

pāpa'i: crab

pau: done; to finish

pau eat: finished eating

pī'āpā: alphabet book

pīkake: jasmine

piko ma'i: genitalia

piko po'o: head

piko waena: umbilicus

pīkoi: tripping weapons

pili: grass

pilikia: trouble, distress

pilina: relationship

Pō: eternity

Pō 'Ōlelo Hawai'i: Hawaiian language night

po'e kahiko: people of old

poepoe: round

pōhaku 'ānai: stone polishers

pōhaku ku'i 'ai: poi pounder

pōhaku 'ulumaika: stones used in a Hawaiian traditional game

pohekula: Asiatic pennywort

pōhinahina: sedge

pohō: damage

poi: pounded taro

poi bowl: fertile place for growing food

pololū: long spear

pono: correct, good, upright, in perfect order

po'o lua: double-headed god

Popoki: lua God

pōpolo: glossy nightshade

pū'iwa: shocked

pulapula: seedling, offspring, descendent

pule: prayer, prayers

pule ho'opau: closing prayer

pule 'ohana: family prayers

pule wehe: opening prayer

punahele: special child

Pūnana Leo: Hawaiian immersion schools

pū'olo: container, bag

pūpū: shells

pu'u: hill

pu'uhonua: places of refuge

pu'upu'u lima: double-fisted god

squid lū'au: dish with squid and leaves of the taro plant

ua ho'omakua ka lā'au: the plant has become a tree

'uala: sweet potato

'uhaloa: small, downy American weed

'uhane: spirit

ula: lobster

ule hala: prop roots of the hala tree

Uli'eo Koa: warrior fitness, preparedness

'ulu: breadfruit
ulu niu: coconut grove
'ulumaika: stones used in a Hawaiian traditional game
'umeke: bowl
'uniki: graduation
'upena: fishing net

wahi pana: legendary place; legendary places
wāhine: women
wāhine kaua: battle women

wai: fresh water
wai huikala: water of purification
wai ola: water and heat therapies
wailele: waterfalls
waiwai: wealth
Wākea: ancestor of the Hawaiian people
wala'au: talking
wana: sea urchin
wao kanaka: agricultural zone
wao nahele: upland forest zone
wauke: paper mulberry tree
wehena: period of discussion

References

Abbott, Isabella Aiona. 1992. *Lāʻau Hawaiʻi: Traditional Hawaiian Uses of Plants*. Honolulu: Bishop Museum Press.

ʻAha Kāne. n.d. "Our Vision, Purpose and Mission." Our Vision, Purpose and Mission: ʻAha Kāne: Ina paʻa ʻole ka pohaku kihi, haʻule ka paia, 2006. Accessed January 13, 2021. https://ahakane.org.

Ahlo, Charles, Jerry Walker, and Rubellite Kawena Johnson. 2000. *Kamehamehaʻs Children Today*. Honolulu, HI: Self-published.

Antonio, Mapuana C. K., Earl S. Hishinuma, Claire Townsend Ing, Fumiaki Hamagami, Adrienne Dillard, B. Puni Kekauoha, Cappy Solatorio, Kevin Cassel, Kathryn L. Braun, and Joseph Keaweʻaimoku Kaholokula. 2020. "A Resilience Model of Adult Native Hawaiian Health Utilizing a Newly Multi-Dimensional Scale." *Behavioral Medicine* 46 (3–4): 258–277. doi:10.1080/0896 4289.2020.1758610.

Auwae, Henry. 2000. Interview with Bonnie Horrigan. Auwae Poʻokela Laʻau Lapaʻau: Master of Hawaiian Medicine. *Alternative Therapies in Health and Medicine* 6 (1): 82–88.

Avendaño, Eleni. 2019. "UH West Oahu Has a New Program in Native Hawaiian Healing." Honolulu Civil Beat, September 5. https://www.civilbeat.org.

Awaiaulu. 2011. "3,000 Volunteers Needed to Bring Historical Hawaiian Language Newspapers to the Internet." *Hawaiʻi Reporter*. November 22. http://www.hawaiireporter.com.

Baclayon, Keoki Kikahi Pai. 2012. "E Ku Makani: A 'Life History' Story of Kahuna Lāʻau Lapaʻau Levon Ohai." Master's thesis, University of Hawaiʻi at Mānoa.

Beckwith, Martha W. 1922. "Hawaiian Riddling." *American Anthropologist* 24 (3): 311–331. doi:10.1525/aa.1922.24.3.02a00030.

Benham, Maenette K. P. 2007. "Moʻōlelo: On Culturally Relevant Story Making from an Indigenous Perspective." In *Handbook of Narrative Inquiry: Mapping a Methodology*, edited by D. Jean Clandinin, 512–534. Thousand Oaks, CA: Sage Publications.

Berger, John. 1994. "Timeline: Hawaiian Entertainment Milestones." *Billboard Newspaper*, April 30. https://books.google.com.

————. 1997. "Island Mele: Jon & Randy Return, with Steve This Time." *Honolulu Star Advertiser,* October 31. http://archives.starbulletin.com.

Blaisdell, Kekuni. 1997. "Historical and Philosophical Aspects of Lapaʻau Traditional Kanaka Maoli Healing Practices." In *Motion Magazine,* November 16. http://www.inmotionmagazine.com.

Braun, Kathryn L., Colette V. Browne, Lana Sue Kaʻopua, Bum Jung Kim, and Noreen Mokuau. 2014. "Research on Indigenous Elders: From Positivistic to Decolonizing Methodologies." *Gerontologist* 54 (1): 117–126.

Braun, Kathryn L., Colette V. Browne, Shelley Muneoka, Tyran Terada, Rachel Burrage, Yan Yan Wu, and Noreen Mokuau. 2021. "Migration and Resilience in Native Hawaiian Elders." *Journal of Ethnic and Cultural Diversity in Social Work* 30 (1–2): 80–103.

Brave Heart, Maria Yellow Horse. 2000. "Wakiksuyapi: Carrying the Historical Trauma of the Lakota." *Tulane Studies in Social Welfare* 21–22: 245–266.

Browne, Colette V., Noreen Mokuau, and Kathryn L. Braun. 2009. "Adversity and Resiliency in the Lives of Native Hawaiian Elders." *Social Work* 54 (3): 253–261. doi:10.1093/sw/54.3.253.

Carlton, Barry S., Deborah A. Goebert, Robin H. Miyamoto, Naleen N. Andrade, Earl S. Hishinuma, George K Makini, Noelle Y. C. Yuen, Cathy K. Bell, Laurie D. McCubbin, Iwalani R. N. Else, et al. 2006. "Resilience, Family Adversity and Well-Being among Hawaiian and Non-Hawaiian Adolescents." *International Journal of Social Psychiatry* 52 (4): 291–308. doi:10.1177/0020764006065136.

Cataluna, Lee. 2019. "Movement to Preserve Heiau Marks 10 Years." *Honolulu Star Advertiser*, November 3. https://www.staradvertiser.com.

Chai, R. Makana Risser. 2005. *Nā Moʻolelo Lomilomi: The Traditions of Hawaiian Massage and Healing*. Honolulu, HI: Bishop Museum Press.

Chun, Malcolm Nāea. 1994. *Must We Wait in Despair: The 1867 Report of the ʻAhahui Lāʻau Lapaʻau of Wailuku, Maui on Native Hawaiian Health*. Honolulu, HI: First People's Productions.

Cook, Bud, Lucia Tarallo-Jensen, Kelley Withy, and Shaun Berry. 2005. "Changes in Kānaka Ma Men's Roles and Health: Healing the Warrior Self." *International Journal of Men's Health* 4 (2): 115–130. doi:10.3149/jmh.0402.115.

Cordy, Ross. 2000. *Exalted Sits the Chief: The Ancient History of Hawaiʻi Island*. Honolulu, HI: Mutual.

Crabbe, Kamanaʻopono M., Mark Eshima, Kealoha Fox, and Keola K. Chan. 2011. *Nā Limahana o Lonopūhā Native Hawaiian Health Consortium*. Honolulu, HI: Office of Hawaiian Affairs. https://www.oha.org.

Crabbe, Kamanaʻopono M., Kealoha Fox, and Holly Kilinahe Coleman. 2017. *Mana Lāhui Kānaka*. Honolulu, HI: Office of Hawaiian Affairs.

Danzan Ryu Ohana. n.d. "ʻOlohe Jerry Walker: Ohana Event Instructor." Accessed January 6, 2021. https://danzanryuohana.wixsite.com.

Daws, Gavan. 1974. *Shoal of Time: A History of the Hawaiian Islands*. Honolulu, HI: University Press of Hawai'i.

DeMattos, Michael. 2016. "'Anakē Lynette Kahekili Kaopuiki Paglinawan: Following in the Steps of Her Ancestors." *Reflections: Narratives of Professional Helping* 21 (2): 49–55. https://reflectionsnarrativesofprofessionalhelping.org.

Desha, Stephen L. 2000. *Kamehameha and His Warrior Kekūhaupi'o*. Translated by Frances N. Frazier. Honolulu, HI: Kamehameha Schools Press.

Donlin, Amanda Lokelani. 2010. "When All the Kāhuna Are Gone: Evaluating Hawai'i's Traditional Hawaiian Healers' Law." *Asian-Pacific Law and Policy Journal* 12 (1): 210–248.

Duponte, Kai, Noreen Mokuau, Tammy Martin, and Lynette Paglinawan. 2010. "'Ike Hawai'i: A Training Program for Working with Native Hawaiians." *Journal of Indigenous Voices in Social Work* 1 (1): 1–24.

Elbert, Samuel H., and Noelani Mahoe. 1970. *Nā Mele o Hawai'i Nei*. Honolulu, HI: University of Hawai'i Press.

Enos, Eric. 2012. "'Aha Kāne—Eric Enos: Working and Caring for the 'Āina." 'Ōiwi TV. https://oiwi.tv.

Ewalt, Patricia L., and Noreen Mokuau. 1995. "Self-Determination from a Pacific Perspective." *Social Work* 40 (2): 168–175.

Eyre, Kawika. 2004. "Suppression of Hawaiian Culture at KS Schools." *Ka'iwakīloumoku, Hawaiian Cultural Center*. January. https://apps.ksbe.edu.

Feher, Joseph, Edward Joesting, and O. A. Bushnell. 1969. *Hawaii: A Pictorial History*. Honolulu, HI: Bishop Museum Press.

Fox, Kealoha K. 2017. "Kūkulu Ola Hou Rebuilding Native Hawaiian Health by Reconnecting Ancestral Practices of Traditional Medicine: An Inventory of Researched Customs, Rituals, and Practices Relating to Hawaiian Ma'i." PhD diss., University of Hawai'i at Mānoa.

Fujita, Ruth, Kathryn L. Braun, and Claire K. Hughes. 2004. "The Traditional Hawaiian Diet: A Review of the Literature." *Pacific Health Dialog* 11 (2): 250–259.

Gillett, Dorothy Kahananui. 1999. *The Queen's Songbook*. Honolulu, HI: Hui Hānai.

Goebert, Deborah, Antonia Alvarez, Naleen N. Andrade, JoAnne Balberde-Kamalii, Barry S. Carlton, Shaylin Chock, Jane J. Chung-Do, et al. 2018. "Hope, Help, and Healing: Culturally Embedded Approaches to Suicide Prevention, Intervention and Postvention Services with Native Hawaiian Youth." *Psychological Services* 15 (3): 332–339. doi:10.1037/ser0000227.

Goodyear-Ka'ōpua, Noelani. 2015. "Reproducing the Ropes of Resistance: Hawaiian Studies Methodologies." In *Kanaka 'Ōiwi Methodologies: Mo'olelo and Metaphor,* edited by Katrina-Ann R. Kapā'anaokalāokeola Nākoa Oliveira and Erin Kahunawaika'ala Wright, 1–29. Honolulu, HI: University of Hawai'i Press.

Gutmanis, June. 1983. *Na Pule Kahiko: Ancient Hawaiian Prayers*. Honolulu, HI: Editions Limited.

———. 1991. *Kahuna Laʻau Lapaʻau*. Honolulu, HI: Island Heritage.

Handy, E. S. Craighill. 1931. *Cultural Revolution in Hawaii*. Honolulu, HI: American Council, Institute of Pacific Relations.

Handy, E. S. Craighill, Kenneth P. Emory, Edwin H. Bryan, Peter H. Buck, and John H. Wise. 1965. *Ancient Hawaiian Civilization: A Series of Lectures Delivered at the Kamehameha Schools*. Rutland, VT: Charles E. Tuttle.

Handy, E. S. Craighill, and Mary Kawena Pukui. 1972. *The Polynesian Family System in Kaʻu, Hawaiʻi*. Rutland, VT: Charles E. Tuttle.

Harvard Health. 2016. "How Music Can Help You Heal." Harvard Health. February 19, 2016. http://www.health.harvard.edu.

Hawaiʻi State Department of Education. n.d. "Hawaiian Language Immersion Program." Accessed January 2, 2021. http://www.hawaiipublicschools.org.

Hawaiʻi State Department of Land and Natural Resources (DLNR). n.d. "Burial Sites Program." Accessed January 3, 2021. http://dlnr.hawaii.gov.

Hewett, Kawaikapuokalani, Cecelia S. Alailima Kawahine, Kuike Kamakea-Ohelo, and Kawena Mann. 2001. "O Ke Aloha Ka Mea I Hoʻola ʻAi—Compassion Is the Healer: An Indigenous Peoples Healing Conference, October 2000, Hawaiʻi." *Pacific Health Dialog* 8 (2): 417–422.

Hiroa, Te Rangi (Sir Peter Buck). 1957. *Arts and Crafts of Hawaii*. Honolulu, HI: Bishop Museum Press.

Ho-Lastimosa, Ilima, Jane J. Chung-Do, Phoebe W. Hwang, Theodore Radovich, Ikaika Rogerson, Kenneth Ho, Samantha Keaulana, Joseph Keaweʻaimoku Kaholokula, and Michael S. Spencer. 2019. "Integrating Native Hawaiian Tradition with the Modern Technology of Aquaponics." *Global Health Promotion* 26 (3): 87–92. doi:10.1177/1757975919831241.

Hoʻomanawanui, Kuʻualoha, Candace Fujikane, Aurora Kagawa-Viviani, Kerry KamakaokaʻIlima Long, and Kekailoa Perry. 2019. "Teaching for Maunakea: Kiaʻi Perspectives." *Amerasia Journal* 45 (2): 271–276. doi:10.1080/00447471.2019.1686318.

Hughes, Claire Kuʻuleilani. 2019. "ʻOpū palaʻai." *Ka Wai Ola,* June 21.

———. 2002. "Look to the Ancestors for Answers." *Ka Wai Ola,* March 1.

Hurley, Timothy. 2021. "Patience ʻPat' Namaka Wiggin Bacon Shared Knowledge of Hawaiian Culture, Traditions." *Honolulu Star Advertiser,* March 21. https://www.staradvertiser.com.

Ii, John Papa. 1983. *Fragments of Hawaiian History*. Honolulu, HI: Bishop Museum Press.

Inglis, Kerri A. 2005. "Kōkua, Mana, and Mālama ʻĀina: Exploring Concepts of Health, Disease, and Medicine in 19th-Century Hawaiʻi." *Hūlili: Multidisciplinary Research on Hawaiian Well-Being* 2 (1): 215–237.

Ka Huli Ao Center for Excellence in Native Hawaiian Law. n.d. "Community Outreach." Accessed January 6, 2021. https://www.law.hawaii.edu.

Kaʻala Farm ʻOhana. 1996. *From Then to Now: A Manual for Doing Things Hawaiian Style*. Honolulu, HI: Short Stack by Native Books.

Kahananui, Dorothy M. 1965. *E Papa-ʻōlelo Kākou (Hawaiian Level One)*. Honolulu: Kamehameha Schools.

Kaholokula, Joseph Keaweʻaimoku, Andrea H. Nacapoy, and Kāʻohimanu Dang. 2009. "Social Justice as a Public Health Imperative for Kānaka Maoli." *AlterNative: An International Journal of Indigenous Peoples* 5 (2): 117–137. doi:10.1177/117718010900500207.

Kamakau, Samuel Manaiakalani. 1961. *Ruling Chiefs of Hawaii*. Honolulu, HI: Kamehameha Schools Press.

———. 1964. *Ka Poʻe Kahiko: The People of Old*. Honolulu, HI: Bishop Museum Press.

———. 1976. *The Works of the People of Old. Na Hana A Ka Poʻe Kahiko*. Honolulu, HI: Bishop Museum Press.

———. 1991. *Tales and Traditions of the People of Old: Nā Moʻolelo a Ka Poʻe Kahiko*. Honolulu, HI: Bishop Museum Press.

Kameʻeleihiwa, Lilikalā. 1992. *Native Land and Foreign Desires: Pehea Lā E Pono Ai?* Honolulu, HI: Bishop Museum Press.

Kanaeokana. n.d. "Ke Kāniwala Aupuni Hawaiʻi Highlights." Accessed January 2, 2021. http://kanaeokana.net/.

Kanahele, George Huʻeu Sanford. 1986. *Kū Kanaka: Stand Tall*. Honolulu, HI: University of Hawaiʻi Press and Waiaha Foundation.

Kāne, Herb Kawainui. 1997. *Ancient Hawaiʻi*. Captain Cook, HI: Kawainui Press.

Koppel, Tom. 1995. *Kanaka: The Untold Story of Hawaiian Pioneers in British Columbia and the Pacific Northwest*. Vancouver, BC: Whitecap Books.

Krauss, Beatrice H. 1993. *Plants in Hawaiian Culture*. Honolulu, HI: University of Hawaiʻi Press.

Laimana Jr., John Kalei. 2011. "The Phenomenal Rise to Literacy in Hawaiʻi: Hawaiian Society in the Early Nineteenth Century." Master's thesis, University of Hawaiʻi at Mānoa.

Lampert, Nicolas. 2013. *A People's Art History of the United States: 250 Years of Activist Art and Artists Working in Social Justice Movements*. New York: The New Press.

Lee, Pali, and Koko Willis. 1987. *Tales from the Night Rainbow*. Honolulu, HI: Paia-Kapela-Willis ʻOhana.

"Lifetime Achievement Award for Hawaiʻinuiākea Dean Osorio." 2019. *University of Hawaiʻi News*. October 28. https://www.hawaii.edu.

Liliʻuokalani, Lydia. 1898. *Hawaii's Story by Hawaii's Queen*. Honolulu, HI: Mutual.

Livable Hawai'i Kai Hui. n.d. "Hawea Heiau complex." Accessed September 30, 2019. https://www.hawaiikaihui.org.

Lopes Jr., Robert Keawe. 2010. "Ka Waihona A Ke Aloha: Ka Papahana Ho'oheno Mele, An Interactive Resource Center for the Promotion, Preservation and Perpetuation of Mele and Mele Practitioners." PhD diss., University of Hawai'i at Mānoa.

Lorenzo-Elarco, J. Hau'oli. 2019. "He Hō'ili'ili Hawai'i: A Brief History of Hawaiian Language Newspapers." Adam Matthew. Sage Publications. April 30. https://www.amdigital.co.uk.

MacKenzie, Melody Kapilialoha. ed. 1991. *Native Hawaiian Rights Handbook*. Honolulu, HI: University of Hawai'i Press.

———. 2015a. "Chapter 1: Historical Background." In *Native Hawaiian Law: A Treatise,* edited by Melody Kapilialoha MacKenzie, Susan K. Serrano, and D. Kapua'ala Sproat, 2–75. Honolulu, HI: Kamehameha.

———. 2015b. "Chapter 2: Public Land Trust." In *Native Hawaiian Law: A Treatise,* edited by Melody Kapilialoha MacKenzie, Susan K. Serrano, and D. Kapua'ala Sproat, 76–146. Honolulu, HI: Kamehameha.

———. 2015c. "Introduction." In *Native Hawaiian Law: A Treatise,* edited by Melody Kapilialoha MacKenzie, Susan K. Serrano, and D. Kapua'ala Sproat, xi–xv. Honolulu, HI: Kamehameha.

MacKenzie, Melody Kapilialoha, Susan K. Serrano, and D. Kapua'ala Sproat, eds. 2015. *Native Hawaiian Law: A Treatise*. Honolulu, HI: Kamehameha.

Malo, David. 1951. *Hawaiian Antiquities: Moolelo Hawaii*. Translated by Nathaniel B. Emerson. Honolulu, HI: Bishop Museum Press.

Miller, Carey D. 1974. "Appendix E: The Influence of Foods and Food Habits upon the Stature and Teeth of the Ancient Hawaiians." In *Early Hawaiians an Initial Study of Skeletal Remains from Mokapu, Oahu,* edited by Charles Snow, 167–175. Lexington: University Press of Kentucky.

Mitchell, Donald D. Kilolani. 2001. *Resource Units in Hawaiian Culture: A Series of Studies Covering Sixteen Important Aspects of Hawaiian Culture*. Rev. ed. Honolulu, HI: Kamehameha Schools Press.

Mokuau, Noreen. 2019. "Ho'oulu." Paper presented at the Myron B. Thompson School of Social Work Meeting of Alumni of Hawaiian Learning Program and Ke A'o Mau, Honolulu, HI, October 2019.

Mokuau, Noreen, Kathryn L. Braun, and Ephrosine Daniggelis. 2012. "Building Family Capacity for Native Hawaiian Women with Breast Cancer." *Health and Social Work* 37 (4): 216–224. doi:10.1093/hsw/hls033.

Mokuau, Noreen, Kamana'opono Crabbe, and Kealoha Fox. 2019. "Kū ka 'Ōhi'a i ka A'ā—'Ōhi'a That Stands amid the Lava Fields." *Hūlili: Multidisciplinary Research on Hawaiian Well-Being* 11 (2): 323–338.

Mokuau, Noreen, Patrick H. DeLeon, Joseph Keaweʻaimoku Kaholokula, Sade Soares, JoAnn U. Tsark, and Coti Haia. 2016. "Challenges and Promise of Health Equity for Native Hawaiians." *National Academy of Medicine (Expert Voices in Health and Health Care),* October, 1–11. https://nam.edu.

Mokuau, Noreen, and Peter Mataira. 2013. "From Trauma to Triumph: Perspectives for Native Hawaiian and Māori peoples." In *Decolonizing Social Work,* edited by Mel Gray, John Coates, Michael Yellow Bird, and Tiani Hetherington, 145–164. Burlington, VT: Ashgate.

Mokuau, Noreen, and Jon Matsuoka. 1995. "Turbulence among a Native People: Social Work Practice with Native Hawaiians." *Social Work* 40 (4): 465–472. doi:10.1093/sw/40.4.465.

Mueller-Dombois, Deiter. 2007. "The Hawaiian Ahupuaʻa Land Use System: Its Biological Resource Zones and the Challenge for Silvicultural Restoration." In *Biology of Hawaiian Streams and Estuaries,* edited by Neal L. Evenhuis and Michael Fitzsimmons, 23–32. Honolulu, HI: Bishop Museum Press.

Nakata, Bob. 1998. "The Struggles of the Waiāhole-Waikāne Community Association." Honolulu, HI. http://www2.hawaii.edu.

Nakuina, Emma Metcalf. 1904. *Hawaii, Its People, Their Legends.* Honolulu, HI: Hawaiʻi Promotion Committee.

Native American Graves Protection and Repatriation Act (NAGPRA). 1990. Pub. L. No. 101–601, 104 Stat. 3048.

Native Hawaiian Health Care Improvement Act. 1988. Pub. L. No. 100–579, 42 USC 11707(9).

Nordyke, Eleanor C. 1989. *The Peopling of Hawaiʻi.* Honolulu, HI: University of Hawaiʻi Press.

Office of Hawaiian Affairs. 2010. *The Disparate Treatment of Native Hawaiians in the Criminal Justice System.* Honolulu, HI: Office of Hawaiian Affairs.

Oliveira, Katrina-Ann R. Kapāʻanaokalāokeola Nākoa. 2019. "Wisdom Maps: Metaphors as Maps." In *Indigenous Education: New Directions in Theory and Practice,* edited by Dawn Zinga, Spencer Lilley, Sandra Styres, and Huia Tomlins-Jahnke, 171–188. Edmonton, Canada: University of Alberta Press.

Osorio, Jon Kay Kamakawiwoʻole. 2014. "Hawaiian Souls: The Movement to Stop the U.S. Military Bombing of Kahoʻolawe." In *A Nation Rising: Hawaiian Movements for Life, Land, and Sovereignty,* edited by Noelani Goodyear-Kaʻopua, Ikaika Hussey, and Erin Kahunawaikaʻala Wright, 137–160. Durham, NC: Duke University Press.

———. 2019. "Hawaiian Studies 478: Mele o ke Hou: Music in Hawaiian Identity." *ScholarSpace.* University of Hawaiʻi at Mānoa. https://scholarspace .manoa.hawaii.edu/.

Paglinawan, Lynette, and Richard Paglinawan. 1991. *Ho'oponopono Conflict Resolution Hawaiian Style.* Unpublished manuscript. Honolulu, HI: In possession of the author.

———. 2012. "Living Hawaiian Rituals: Lua, Ho'oponopono, and Social Work." *Hūlili: Multidisciplinary Research on Hawaiian Well-Being* 8 (1): 1–18.

Paglinawan, Lynette K., Richard Likeke Paglinawan, Dennis Kauahi, and Valli Kalei Kanuha. 2020. *Nānā I Ke Kumu,* Vol. 3. Honolulu, HI: Lili'uokalani Trust.

Paglinawan, Richard Kekumuikawaiokeola, Mitchell Eli, Moses Kalauokalani Elwood, and Jerry Walker. 2006. *Lua: Art of the Hawaiian Warrior.* Honolulu, HI: Bishop Museum Press.

Paik, Kaleo. 2009. "Hawea." In *Hoi Mai Ka Lei i Mamo: Poems by Kaleo Paik.* Honolulu, HI: Self-published.

———. 2013. "Kunia." In *Hoi Mai Ka Lei i Mamo: Poems by Kaleo Paik.* Honolulu, HI: Self-published.

Pang, Gordon Y. K. 2007. "Reburial of Stored Hawaiian Iwi Sought." *Honolulu Advertiser,* April 12. http://the.honoluluadvertiser.com.

Polynesian Voyaging Society. n.d. "Hawaiian Lunar Month." Hawaiian Voyaging Traditions. Accessed December 28, 2020. http://archive.hokulea.com.

Proceedings of the Constitutional Convention of Hawai'i of 1978. 1980. Vol. 1. Honolulu, HI: State of Hawai'i.

Pukui, Mary Kawena. 1983. *'Ōlelo No'eau: Hawaiian Proverbs and Poetical Sayings.* Honolulu, HI: Bishop Museum Press.

Pukui, Mary Kawena, and Samuel H. Elbert. 1986. *Hawaiian Dictionary.* Honolulu, HI: University of Hawai'i Press.

Pukui, Mary Kawena, E. W. Haertig, and Catherine A. Lee. 1972. *Nānā I Ke Kumu (Look to the Source).* Vol. 1. Honolulu, HI: Hui Hānai.

Pukui, Mary Kawena, E. W. Haertig, Catherine A. Lee, and John F. McDermott. 1979. *Nānā I Ke Kumu (Look to the Source).* Vol. 2. Honolulu, HI: Hui Hānai.

Roig, Suzanne. 2006. "Six Honored This Year as Living Treasures." *Honolulu Advertiser,* Jan. 22, 2006. http://the.honoluluadvertiser.com.

Saleebey, Dennis, ed. 1997. *The Strengths Perspective in Social Work Practice.* 2nd ed. White Plains, NY: Longman.

Shore, Bradd. 1989. "Mana and Tapu." In *Developments in Polynesian Ethnology,* edited by Robert Borofsky and Alan Howard, 151–186. Honolulu, HI: University of Hawai'i Press.

Snow, Charles E. 1974. *Early Hawaiians an Initial Study of Skeletal Remains from Mokapu, Oahu.* Lexington: University Press of Kentucky.

Sodetani, Naomi. 2003. "Way of the Warrior." *Hana Hou! The Magazine of Hawaiian Airlines,* April–May 2003. https://hanahou.com.

Spencer, Michael, and Mary Oneha. 2019. Waimanalo Health Center. Waimanalo, HI. Video. https://vimeo.com.

Sproat, D. Kapuaʻala. 2015. "From Wai to Kānāwai: Water Law in Hawaiʻi." In *Native Hawaiian Law: A Treatise,* edited by Melody Kapilialoha MacKenzie, Susan K. Serrano, and D. Kapuaʻala Sproat, 522–610. Honolulu, HI: Kamehameha.

Summers, Catherine C. 1990. *Hawaiian Cordage.* Honolulu, HI: Bishop Museum Press.

Thompson, Christina. 2019. *Sea People: The Puzzle of Polynesia.* New York: Harper Collins Publisher.

Thrum, Thomas G. 1907. *Hawaiian Folk Tales: A Collection of Native Legends.* London: Lakeside.

Trust for Public Land. n.d. "Hawea Heiau Complex and Keawawa Wetland." Accessed January 3, 2021. https://www.tpl.org.

Tsark, JoAnn, Kekuni Blaisdell, and Noa Emmett Aluli. 1998. "The Health of Native Hawaiians." Special issue, *Pacific Health Dialog: Journal of Community Health and Clinical Medicine for the Pacific* 5 (2): 228–404.

Weber, Bret A., and Amanda Wallace. 2018. "Revealing the Empowerment Revolution: A Literature Review of the Model Cities Program." *Journal of Urban History* 38 (1): 173–192.

Wesley-Esquimaux, Cynthia C., and Magdalena Smolewski. 2004. *Historical Trauma and Aboriginal Healing.* Ottawa, Ontario: The Aboriginal Healing Foundation.

Wilcox, Leslie. 2011. "Claire Hughes." May 3, 2011. *Long Story Short with Leslie Wilcox.* Visual podcast, 26:52. https://www.pbshawaii.org.

Williams, Julie Stewart. 1993. "Kamehameha the Great." Honolulu, HI: Kamehameha Schools Press.

Wilson, William, and Kauanoe Kamanā. 2006. "'For the Interest of the Hawaiians Themselves': Reclaiming the Benefits of Hawaiian-Medium Education." *Hūlili: Multidisciplinary Research on Hawaiian Well-Being* 3 (1): 150–182.

Wu, Yan Yan, Kathryn L. Braun, Alvin T. Onaka, Brian Y. Horiuchi, Caryn J. Tottori, and Lynne Wilkens. 2017. "Life Expectancies in Hawaiʻi: A Multi-ethnic Analysis of 2010 Tables." *Hawaiʻi Journal of Medicine and Public Health* 76 (1): 9–14. https://www.ncbi.nlm.nih.gov.

Van Dyke, Jon M. 2008. *Who Owns the Crown Lands of Hawaiʻi?* Honolulu, HI: University of Hawaiʻi Press.

Yamane, David P., Steffen G. Oeser, and Jill Omori. 2010. "Health Disparities in the Native Hawaiian Homeless." *Hawaiʻi Medical Journal* 69 (6): 35–41. https://www.ncbi.nlm.nih.gov.

Young, Kanalu. n.d. "Pule No Ke Ea: Prayer for Sovereignty." *Ulukau Collection.* Accessed December 28, 2020. http://www.ulukau.org/.

Index

About the Authors and the Photographer

NOREEN KEHAULANI MOKUAU is a descendent of Ka-leo-puupuu-a-ka-uaua and Kaui-o-kalaninaleimaumau Kana'e on her father's side and Kahele and Sentaro Ishii on her mother's side. She has been known to begin speeches by sharing her genealogy and the influence of family and place on her work. In these "talks," she will often say that all members of her family— past, present, and future—stand with her in the sharing of stories and information. She believes that our ancestral past holds deep reservoirs of information that can benefit people today and tomorrow. As the first Native Hawaiian woman with a doctorate in social work and the first Native Hawaiian dean of a school of social work and public health, she is committed to education that is anchored in excellence and founded in the unique attributes of Hawai'i and the Pacific-Asia region. As a professor emerita with nearly forty years of service at the University of Hawai'i at Mānoa Thompson School of Social Work & Public Health, she continues to be committed to social justice and health equity. By its nature, her work is rooted in the 'ohana (family) and community and framed in cultural essence. As with all things in Hawaiian culture, there is appreciation and acknowledgement of the pilina (relationships) of people, land, and spiritual realm.

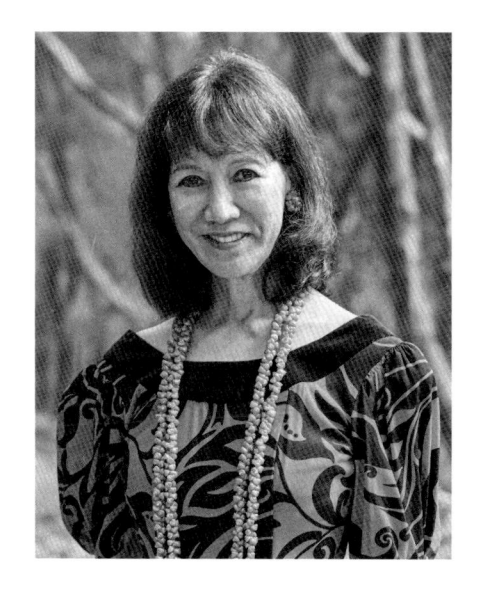

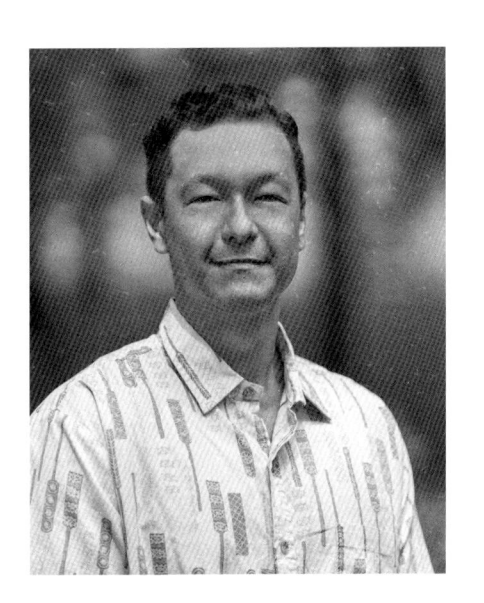

SHAYNE KUKUNAOKALĀ YOSHIMOTO is a pulapula (seedling, offspring, descendent) of Keahinuimakahahaikalani Kuhihewa laua ʻo Wahineaea Keikiomeheula Lililehua Kamaikaumaka of Ualapuʻe, Molokaʻi, with family ties to Maui, and to Papakōlea, Oʻahu. Having obtained his undergraduate and graduate degrees from the University of Hawaiʻi at Mānoa, his professional journey has led him back to the UHM Thompson School of Social Work & Public Health. His career includes four years with the Honolulu Community Action Program, providing services to vulnerable populations in Kahaluʻu and Palolo, and three years with Hui Mālama O Ke Kai as the ʻOhana Program specialist tasked with developing culturally anchored programming for families in the Waimānalo community. He currently serves as the executive director at Blueprint for Change, a nonprofit that provides the fiscal, administrative, and technical support to a statewide system of Neighborhood Places that address prevention services for families at risk of child abuse and neglect. He is a founding co-instructor and coordinator of Ke Aʻo Mau, a cultural course at the Thompson School of Social Work & Public Health. His cultural foundation provides a unique lens that informs his personal and professional life. He believes that the restoration of Native Hawaiian spiritual structures, cosmology, and healing practices will greatly benefit the overall health and well-being of the lāhui (Hawaiian nation).

KATHRYN LENZNER BRAUN is professor of public health and social work and the Barbara Cox Anthony Endowed Chair in Aging at the University of Hawai'i at Mānoa. She serves as graduate chair for the PhD in public health, teaching courses in systematic review, research design, qualitative methods, and evaluation. She also heads the Hā Kūpuna National Resource Center for Native Hawaiian Elders at the UHM Thompson School of Social Work & Public Health, and works with the John A. Burns School of Medicine on projects to improve interdisciplinary geriatric care and support research to reduce health disparities in Hawai'i. She has lived in Hawai'i for more than forty years, earning both her

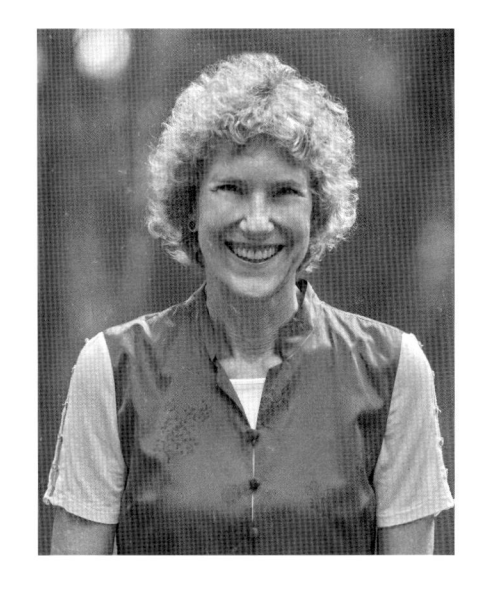

master's and doctoral degrees in public health from UHM. Prior to her hire as a faculty member at UHM in 1993, she worked with Catholic Charities Hawai'i providing services to the elderly in Chinatown, Kalihi, and Palama, and then for ten years with the Queen's Medical Center evaluating programs designed to improve elder care and increase patient safety. Past research with Native Hawaiians includes five years with the Pacific Diabetes Resource Center and eighteen years with the 'Imi Hale Native Hawaiian Cancer Network. She is named for (and much idolized) her paternal grandmother, Ruth Lenzner Braun.

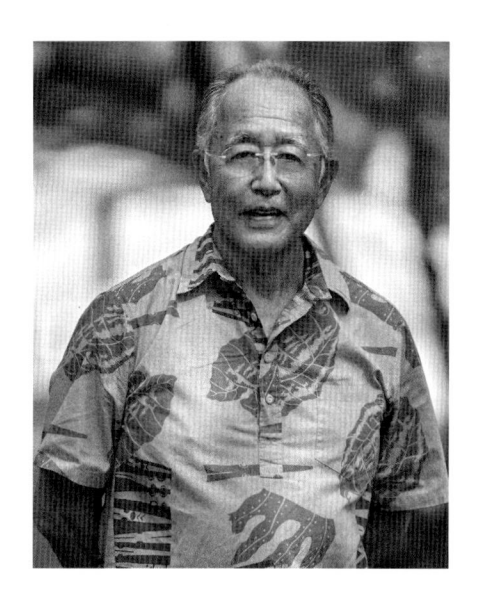

SHUZO UEMOTO is a respected photographer of exacting and timeless portraiture that captures and distills a myriad of nuances and moods. Further, his portraiture is known for its cultural and spiritual sensitivities, as seen in his personal work and in the two volumes of *Nānā I Na Loea Hula—Look to the Hula Resources* (1984) published by the Kalihi-Palama Culture and Arts Society. He has lived in Hawai'i since 1953. His interest in photography began in college. He has worked as the principal photographer for the Honolulu Museum of Art for the past twenty-three years and as lecturer in photography at Kapi'olani Community College since 1988. He has exhibited his works at local, national, and international venues, including Hawai'i and the continental United States; Paris, France; and Osaka, Japan. His work is included in private collections, as well as at the Honolulu Museum of Art and the Hawai'i State Foundation on Culture and the Arts. His published works can be found in *Contemporary Photographers of Hawai'i* (1985); *American Photographer* (1981–1987); *Nānā I Na Loea Hula* vols. 1 and 2 (1984 and 1997); and *Lessons of Aloha with Brother Noland* (1999). He is listed in the *Index to American Photographic Collections* by the International Museum of Photography at the George Eastman House in New York.